The Rhetoric of Breast Cancer

Lexington Studies in Health Communication

Series Editors: Leandra H. Hernández and Kari Nixon

National and international governments have recognized the importance of widespread, timely, and effective health communication, as research shows that accurate, patient-centered, and culturally competent health communication can improve patient and community health care outcomes. This interdisciplinary series examines the role of health communication in society and is receptive to manuscripts and edited volumes that use a variety of theoretical, methodological, interdisciplinary, and intersectional approaches. We invite contributions on a variety of health communication topics including but not limited to health communication in a digital age; race, gender, ethnicity, class, physical abilities, and health communication; critical approaches to health communication; feminisms and health communication; LGBTQIA health; interpersonal health communication perspectives; rhetorical approaches to health communication; organizational approaches to health communication; health campaigns, media effects, and health communication; multicultural approaches to health communication; and international health communication. This series is open to contributions from scholars representing communication, women's and gender studies, public health, health education, discursive analyses of medical rhetoric, and other disciplines whose work interrogates and explores these topics. Successful proposals will be accessible to an interdisciplinary audience, advance our understanding of contemporary approaches to health communication, and enrich our conversations about the importance of health communication in today's health landscape.

Titles in the Series

The Rhetoric of Breast Cancer: Patient-to-Patient Discourse in an Online Community, by Carie S. Tucker King

The Rhetoric of Breast Cancer

Patient-to-Patient Discourse in an Online Community

Carie S. Tucker King

LEXINGTON BOOKS
Lanham • Boulder • New York • London

Published by Lexington Books
An imprint of The Rowman & Littlefield Publishing Group, Inc.
4501 Forbes Boulevard, Suite 200, Lanham, Maryland 20706
www.rowman.com

Unit A, Whitacre Mews, 26-34 Stannary Street, London SE11 4AB

British Library Cataloguing in Publication Information Available

Library of Congress Cataloging-in-Publication Data Available

ISBN 978-1-4985-5244-8 (cloth : alk. paper)
ISBN 978-1-4985-5245-5 (electronic)

∞™ The paper used in this publication meets the minimum requirements of American National Standard for Information Sciences Permanence of Paper for Printed Library Materials, ANSI/NISO Z39.48-1992.

Printed in the United States of America

This work is dedicated to my mother Suzanne, who transparently shares her experiences with me, and to the 1 in 8 American women who will be diagnosed with breast cancer during their lifetimes.

Table of Contents

Introduction

Nothing can prepare a woman to hear, "You have breast cancer." In fact, in the foreword of *The Breast: Comprehensive Management of Benign and Malignant Diseases*, Dr. LaSalle D. Leffall, Jr. (Professor of Surgery at Howard University Hospital and Past President of both the American Cancer Society and the American College of Surgeons) writes,

> There are some experiences that are so profound that those who have shared them are in some ways estranged from those who haven't. Such is often the case in women who have confronted breast cancer—a diagnosis that usually evokes fear and major concern among patients, their families, and other loved ones. . . .
>
> When speaking about breast cancer, surgeons speak about giving patients hope, not some unrealistic hope but one that is realistic, because almost always there is something that can be done to make patients better. When we grant patients hope, we grant them one of the greatest of all human joys, and that is the joy of anticipation—that perhaps just maybe, there is something that can be done to help them. (Leffall, 1998, p. xvii)

Patients who are diagnosed with breast cancer need hope. And although they may search for that hope in the voices of their healthcare providers—e.g., their surgeons, oncologists, nurses, and technicians—patients also search for hope in the voices of those who have gone before them: those who have conquered the disease and the challenges that come with it. Patients who confront breast cancer need hope because, although the disease is not a death sentence, the diagnosis continues to bring potentially painful, challenging, and unanticipated complications like damaging treatments, amputation, re-construction, nausea, changed taste buds and cravings, hair and nail loss, financial drain, and a fear of the unknown. The diagnosis also brings about confusing thoughts and questions about self-identity, medical treatments and finances, symbols like pink ribbons, and words like "survivor" and "battle."

My research into what I call the "rhetoric of breast cancer" began in 2008, when my mother was diagnosed with the disease. Being a medical editor at the time and having worked in surgery and women's health, I determined to know everything I could about breast cancer so I could advocate on Mom's behalf. As I researched and began to see the hope that patients shared with each other, I began to study patient discourses in online spaces. Now, almost a decade later, I seek to listen to and to prioritize the voices of women who are diagnosed with breast cancer and to learn about their perspectives of the disease process (diagnosis, treatment, and recovery) and about the patient experience—because *patient voices matter*. These patients speak because they seek change, advocacy, unity, and hope.

The experience of cancer today differs from my grandmother's experience with gynecologic cancer and, more specifically, with my great aunt's experience with breast cancer. In the 1970s, my great aunt underwent surgery for the simple biopsy of a breast mass. After surgery, she awoke to find that she had undergone a radical mastectomy—that is, because her cancer was more advanced than her physicians anticipated, her breast tissue for the breast with the tumor as well as her chest muscle under the affected breast and the sentinel lymph nodes under that arm were removed (a modified Halsted mastectomy). She underwent the procedure without giving consent and thus without having a say in her care. Once she recovered from the surgical procedure, she creatively expanded her physical therapy: she purchased paint and paint brushes and went to work painting the exterior of her brick house, rehabilitating the arm affected by the mastectomy and recovering much of her ability to move.

Of course, care at that time was more extreme than care is today because breast surgeons and oncologists knew less and had fewer options (Wagner, Martin, and Bland, 1998, p. 12). (Historic treatments included removal of the tumor, breast, skin, pectoral muscles, and axillary nodes followed by cauterization or wash or spray of a carbolic-acid solution [Wagner, Martin, and Bland, 1998, pp. 1–9].) In the early 20th century, standard therapy for mid-stage to advanced breast cancer continued to be the Halsted mastectomy, during which the surgeon removed all tissue related to the breast to ensure that all potentially cancerous cells were removed: "[W]e regularly clean out the infraclavicular and usually the supraclavicular region and remove a part, at least, of the pectoralis major muscle" (Halstead, 1894, p. 497). The Halsted mastectomy, considered revolutionary in its time, required that the surgery be conducted with the tissues removed in one piece to decrease infection (Wagner, Martin, and Bland, 1998, p. 11). This therapy was dismembering, leaving the patients scarred and sometimes unable to use their arms naturally or to move comfortably or easily; their lives were riddled with complications from treatments that were proven most effective for the most extreme cases of breast cancer (Keränen, 2010, pp. 38–39). As researchers learned more about breast cancer, surgeons investigated new treatments and therapies that were less extreme, responding to an obvious medical need and to the voices of women who demanded less extreme therapy for earlier stages of cancer (Keränen, 2010, pp. 39). As radiation, hormonal therapy, and chemotherapy treatments; diagnostic tests like mammography, interventional radiology, and ultrasonography; and multimodal therapy have been integrated into the treatment of breast cancer, care has become more diverse and customized per a patient's diagnosis (Wagner, Martin, and Bland, 1998, pp. 12–16).

Women's health and medical concerns are currently part of ongoing national debate of women's healthcare, and women's voices are vital in defining those issues and concerns. Women's voices should be prioritized in considering their health concerns—to allow them to serve as advocates "to gain access to or influence the power structures that surround health, wellness, illness, safety, medical testing, diagnosis, prognosis, hospitalization, and treatments" (White-Farnham, Finer, and Molloy, 2017). Women's voices are an important part of the medical discourse around breast cancer. Their voices have become more unified in the last forty years—through large nonprofits that focus on research, media that covers issues and developments related to the disease, fundraising efforts, unifying symbols and marketing, face-to-face support meetings, and online support groups and communities where members can converse to gain information and to share their experiences. Their voices have altered the surgical and medical treatment for the disease; the treatments, however, continue to alter patients' lives in ways that only experiential evidence can prove and only illness narratives can fully elucidate.

Although breast cancer is less of a mystery than it was when my great aunt underwent surgery, cancer is cancer, and we still shudder at the sound of the word. We know more, but we are surrounded by a plethora of information, some confusing, overwhelming, and frightening, particularly for a patient who has just heard, "You have cancer."

Information was a challenge for my mother when she was diagnosed with cancer. She was overwhelmed with all of the possibilities: when she was originally diagnosed, her breast surgeon provided her with a canvas bag that contained ten books and a stack of brochures about nutrition, psychological care, wigs, prosthetics, possible side effects, options, and other data. She also struggled to control information. Her friends asked about her diagnosis and treatment, and, although she appreciated their caring, she began to feel like she had no control, specifically of her medical information. She was particularly embarrassed when several concerned friends asked in a public place about her breast (a private body part and sex organ), her surgery, and the disease and its side effects. To protect her, my father and I created a blog where she could control the information she released: she could share what she wanted when and with whom she wanted. She could also control her energy and her time and blog when she did not feel weak, sick, or tired. As she blogged about her experiences, my mother found writing to be therapeutic, and later, she published her blog as a book that journals her cancer experience (Tucker, 2010). She has taken her writing further to serve as a resource for many other women who have been diagnosed with breast cancer and, looking for help, have contacted her.

I read the information that the healthcare providers gave my mother, but I also began to search for additional sources, particularly experiential information from women who had confronted breast cancer. In my search for information, I found Breastcancer.org: an online source that hosts a community of men and women diagnosed with breast cancer. The community became a valuable source of information as well as an inspiration for me. In the information pages and discussion board of this online community, I found credible information about breast cancer, framed by patient perspectives and narrative focused on survival, wellness, and life. These voices empowered me to advocate and study to help take care of my mother.[1] Once she completed treatment, I stopped visiting Breastcancer.org as a registered member and accessed only the non-password-protected (public) areas to learn through virtual ethnography and to obtain "a greater understanding of human action" (Segal, 2005, p. 2) through rhetorical and discourse analysis. (I altered my role in the online community and obtained institutional review board [IRB] approval for my research to ensure ethical practices in my data collection and analysis. I will address these ethical dilemmas in chapter 4.)

The result is this book, which is for a variety of readers:

- communication and language scholars who study the rhetorics of health and medicine,
- information architects who design the frameworks for online communities,
- healthcare providers who seek to know what patients discuss in large online communities,
- investigators who apply the methods of virtual ethnography and rhetorical and discourse analyses to their data,
- theorists who want to better understand trends in communication and patient discourse, and
- researchers and ethicists who consider standards for the ethical investigation of discourse in online communities.

Various other unanticipated audiences will be interested in what I call the *rhetoric of breast cancer*.

The rhetoric of breast cancer is the use of language for interaction in the community of those who have been diagnosed with breast cancer and are communicating about their experiences. This discourse includes patients' illness narratives as well as discussions about related experiences, resources they have found, and other elements of life that their disease affects, and it resounds with the unified voice of the community. However, specific posts contain elements that reflect important and unique characteristics of individual members and their messages as well as the post in which the discourse exists. Specifically, on Breastcancer.org, members share their illness narratives about breast cancer and thus use language in a unique way—with meaning, context, and tone—that relates specifically to the disease or to other experiences that the community members are sharing. (Chapter 2 specifically addresses the characteristics of the rhetoric of breast cancer.)

FOUNDATIONS IN THE RHETORICS OF HEALTH AND MEDICINE

The term "rhetoric" was created by Aristotle, the Greek scholar and teacher who sought to define public speaking in the established situations of forensic, epideictic, and deliberative speaking (Aristotle, 1924/350 B.C.E., Bk. I, Pt. 3, paras. 1–4; Lawson-Tancred, 2004, p. 17). However, as communication analysis has proceeded past this traditional definition, theorists and rhetoricians have expanded the concept to incorporate language into other circumstances and thus in other fields and situations. "On Aristotle's criteria . . . there can be many instances of rhetorical argument that fall under none of the three kinds of rhetoric" (Garver, 2009, p. 4). Whereas the use of language for persuasion may originally been identified to have "only three objectives: the establishment of justice of its given subject-matter . . . of its admirability or . . . of its advisability" (Lawson-Tancred, 2004, p. 17), changes in society, economics, politics, technology, and other fields have influenced our perception and thus definition of rhetoric.

As our perception of rhetoric shifts, the application of rhetorical theory in regard to narrative and discourse is expanding to include new contexts, audiences, and fields of practice. Today, theorists show that the definition has changed "to include the theory of both production and reception of texts, both spoken and written, and it has moved well beyond its original applications in public speaking to include more generally the persuasive element in all human interaction" (Derkatch and Segal, 2005, p. 138). Instead of being categorized into Aristotle's static categories, rhetoric has expanded to accomplish different purposes and to reflect the reality in which it exists:

> For rhetoric as such is not rooted in any past condition of human society. It is rooted in an essential function of language itself, a function that is wholly

> realistic, and is continually born anew; the use of language as a symbolic means of inducing cooperation in beings that by nature respond to symbols. (Burke, 1969, p. 43)

Rhetoric then is a cooperative act: "[T]he act of identification itself, in which the rhetor and the audience, having overcome their 'division,' *act together*" (Segal, 2005, p. 12). This cooperative act allows for "alternative discursive practices" (Hiefferon and Brown, 2000, p. 247) in various fields, including communication related to wellness, fitness, nutrition, diagnoses, and medicine (which includes complementary and alternative medicine [e.g., Ben-Arye, Traube, Schachter, et al., 2010; Derkatch, 2012; Derkatch, 2015]). Traditionally, this communication was produced and interpreted by medical professionals (Bellwoar, 2005, p. 325), who were the subject-matter experts, and by empowered patients (Segal, 2009, p. 352) then accepted and responded to the communication, making decisions from this communication (in various forms, including print and digital texts, discourse, and visual rhetoric). This communication is important in the investigation of language as it relates to medicine. It is also important to research as scholars investigate language in medicine and science as well as the rhetorical and discourse-focused methods that these scholars use:

> Our field also uses an extensive repertoire of methodological approaches, in particular developing our own combination of ethnographic studies of the workplace and textual analyses. Again, that is an important interdisciplinary contribution because no other field seeks so persistently to uncover the constitutive relations between the details of language and the description of content and context in medicine. . . . [O]ur field brings the potential for valuable contributions to the knowledge and analysis of the discourses of medicine; research with a growing impact on the medical profession and its education and practice. (Barton, 2005, p. 248)

Thus, we have established the field of rhetorics of health and medicine (as labeled by Scott, Segal, and Keränen, 2013).

As the field emerges and expands, researchers in the field are charged to consider "health texts, artifacts, genres, and practices" and other "rhetorics that influence daily life and public meanings and practices" (Scott, Segal, and Keränen, 2013, p. 2). Already established and influential studies of these rhetorics include communication research related to atherosclerosis (Mol, 2002); counterpublics to "National Breast Cancer Awareness Month" (Pezzullo, 2003); breastfeeding (Koerber, 2005); obesity and weight-loss surgery (Throsby, 2007); counter-narratives to disability (Barton, 2007); biology (to teach microscopy; Dinolfo, Heifferon, and Temesvari, 2007); intersex communities (Still, 2008); Severe Acute Respiratory Syndrome (SARS; Ding, 2009); fibromyalgia (Graham, 2009); pandemic flu (and related metaphors;

Angeli, 2012); choice related to menstruation and contraception (Woods, 2012); and diabetes (Arduser, 2017). These studies make "interdisciplinary contributions" that help "medicine and health care gain a more contextualized understanding of their practices of professionalism in language" (Barton, 2005, p. 246). They expand the rhetorics of health and medicine and establish the value of these discourses within health and medical practices and research.

The persuasive element of rhetoric as it relates to health and medicine has become more flexible, as most stakeholders in many medical scenarios are communicating to persuade: e.g., patients who are ill presenting their symptoms as evidence of disease to their healthcare providers; physicians persuading patients to partner to choose a treatment and then to comply and follow the prescribed regimen; clinical and laboratory researchers proposing research projects as they seek to fund and to publish their investigations; medical sales and pharmaceutical representatives selling products and prescription drugs to the market; surgeons and specialists assuring family members and extending hope; and allied-health and nursing professionals and technicians gathering evidence for physicians and/or persuading patients to follow instructions. Persuasion occurs in a variety of locations, such as in the medical office, the clinic, the surgical suite, the laboratory, and the hospital waiting room. The rhetorics of health and medicine have focused on the scholarly study of these persuasive interactions, with researchers studying documentation, visual elements, "emerging and hybrid genres," discussions between healthcare providers and patients on various topics that have legal implications, documentation of patients' and physicians' legal and ethical responsibilities, and other discourse (Haas, 2009, p. 210). The call for flexible research of other discourse encourages theorists to consider nontraditional texts that fit into the medical context.

These changes, shifts, and expansions in rhetoric and the recognition of the rhetorics of health and medicine align with the changes in how people access and manage information; technology has changed the way people, particularly adults in the United States and first-world countries, find information. Their use of technology is becoming common activity and thus fits into the call to consider "rhetorics that influence daily life and public meanings and practices" (Scott, Segal, and Keränen, 2013, p. 2). Online access to information is as common as are the smart phones that most Americans own and use throughout the day, and health and information is becoming more accessible and acceptable. For example, 59 percent of U.S. adult Internet users have searched for health information online in the past year (Fox and Duggan, 2013, para. 8), and 35 percent self-report that they have used Internet sources to self-diagnose or to diagnose someone else's medical issues (Fox and Duggan, 2013, para. 1). Healthcare professionals continue to be the primary source of medical information for "serious health episodes" and for health-related information, although 70 percent of U.S. adults gather information or care from a provider, 60 percent obtain information or support from family members or friends, and 24 percent accept information or support from patients who have the same diagnosis (Fox and Duggan, 2013, para. 7).

Rhetoric and communication scholars recognize this shift in information management and are considering digital texts, analyzing what they contain, considering how audiences and subject-matter experts interact in digital spaces, and identifying how communication experts are becoming part of interdisciplinary projects to help medical experts better communicate via technology (Koerber and Still, 2008). For this reason, we must consider the rhetorics of health and medicine as a still-emerging field (Meloncon and Frost, 2015), and perhaps one of the most exciting calls for our field is to allow a diverse blend of voices and perspectives to discuss health and medicine (*Present Tense* Editors, 2012).

PATIENT VOICES AND DISCOURSE IN THE RHETORICS OF HEALTH AND MEDICINE

Traditionally, in the medical setting, the patient exists "primarily in relation to the role of the physician" and is "a construct of the physician" (Segal, 2005, p. 37). Thus, the patient has been included in the rhetorics of health and medicine but frequently has had a role that depends on the professionally trained provider. However, their relationship is interactive, and both stakeholders (the patient and the physician) are audiences to each other. As a result, a majority of our studies have focused on the exchange of information within medical settings that are related to professionals in the medical field, such as the interaction in a physician's office during a physician-and-patient interview (Segal, 2005, pp. 37–58). The value of this encounter is the exchange of information: the patient presents an invisible complaint and shares narrative about his/her experiences and symptoms, and the physician then creates a view that is "clinically important" (Segal, 2005, p. 40). The discourse between the physician and patient values the voice of the patient, who is sharing information that, framed in the circumstances, presents an illness narrative. Thus, the patient's story is framed with descriptions of symptoms, experiences, treatments, and limitations, and the patient's narrative is a part of the construction of medical knowledge (Segal, 2005, p. 48). This construction comes from studying the culture of patient narratives as if studying per sociology or anthropology, using research methods that are typically affiliated with the social sciences such as ethnography (see Wilce, 2009, p. 201) and qualitative methods such as narrative and content analysis (see Bury, 2001, p. 281).

Keränen (2010) focuses on the patient's role in her analysis of rhetoric related to Datagate and the case of fraudulent patient enrollment for the National Surgical Adjuvant Breast and Bowel Project (NSABP). Patients who volunteered in breast-cancer research through the NSABP felt victimized after the *Chicago Tribute* published a front-page story exposing that physicians involved in the NSABP were fraudulent in their methods to enroll patients. These patients and their advocates responded by meeting together and by testifying in the case, thus seeking to call their providers to accountability and to elevate the patients' voices. Keränen (2010) analyzes patient communication with that shared purpose:

> Although their [the women's] voices formed a powerful core of complaints, in the decade before blogs and message boards came to dominate public life, much of the vernacular rhetoric about Datagate—the everyday communication that occurred around water coolers, over phone lines, or in support groups—is lost to history, so one of the challenges I faced in this study was to represent women's concerns without replicating the silencing of, or the speaking for, women that occurred as the controversy progressed. . . . Their voices reveal the dilemmas of stakeholder exclusion from and inclusion in the research process, illuminating how the scientific endeavor is helped and hindered by more voices. But these voices also provide the opportunity to understand what happened at a moment when women felt compelled to contribute to the broader controversy over research that affected their lives. (p. 120)

Keränen seeks to value the patients' voices as they relate to this case, particularly because the patients' discourses related to the situation were not recorded and retained.

Seigel (2013) also values "patient voices" in her rhetorical analysis of pregnancy manuals. She elevates the pregnant woman to "user" and thus to a vital part of the medical community—the individuals who are "using" the services and medical information that healthcare providers publish in these manuals (Seigel, 2013, p. 22). She addresses the changes in the medical model and acknowledges that women can be engaged in managing their care as equal partners. Seigel (2013) seeks to redefine women's contributions to technical communication and writing about science (p. 8) by applying feminist theory and standards established in previous studies (e.g., Koerber, 2005; Owens, 2009) and thus categorizing pregnancy manuals in the same way (Seigel, 2013, p. 8). In her own way, Seigel also elevates the voice of the patient by speaking in first person in her first chapter, sharing personal testimony and the motivation behind her study. In this way, she, the "user," becomes a part of the narrative as recipient of care *and* scholar who is analyzing the rhetorics of health and medicine.

The designation of rhetorics of health and medicine will continue to grow as we "push boundaries," as we have been challenged:

> We also need to consider engagement with different types of evidence, communities, patients, and other active participants in healthcare, and we need to determine ways to move the work we do across disease domains. Both of these push the established boundaries, but if accomplished will allow the field to have an impact. (Meloncon and Frost, 2015, p. 11)

This charge encourages scholars to consider the stakeholders and the communication related to health and medicine and to consider new dimensions that provide diverse perspectives. These perspectives are introduced in Mol's (2002) *The Body Multiple: Ontology in Medical Practice*, when she addresses these perspectives and perspectivalism:

> Like patients, or so it is said, doctors have a *perspective*. They attribute meaning to what happens to bodies and lives. Even though doctors interpret the bodies and lives of others, whereas patients talk primarily about their own.
>
> Perspectivalism turns doctors and patients into equals, for both interpret the world they live in. But to say this is also to reinforce their division, because the interpretations doctors and patients give must differ, linked as they are to the specific history, interests, roles, and horizons of each group. In perspectivalism, the words "disease" and "illness" are no longer used to contrast physical facts with personal meaning. Instead, they differentiate between the perspectives of doctors on the one hand and those of patients on the other. (pp. 10–11)

Mol's explanation creates a balance between the perspectives of physicians and patients and thus justifies equalization of their voices, as partners in decision-making but also as separate speakers in the medical arena, because their different experiences and perspectives of the same circumstances matter. She also gives the patient ownership of the bodies and lives that make health and medicine necessary; in fact, the existence of patients justifies the existence of the rhetorics of health and medicine: without the patient's body, life, fitness, nutrition, illness, experience, issues, and needs, medicine would not exist, and thus the field that focuses on the rhetorics of health and medicine would not exist.

Meloncon and Frost (2015) further challenge rhetorical scholars to creatively consider discourses related to the rhetorics of health and medicine and to consider the every-day exchanges that are foundational in the discourses of this field:

> For many years, an often-looked aspect of health and medicine was the communicative dimension, that is the discourses—oral, written, visual, and technological. When we speak of discourses, we are thinking about lab notes, case reports, electronic medical records, patient notes, regulatory documents, insurance claims, online health information, patient education materials, and pharmaceutical advertisements, to name a few. Because of its everydayness, the

> written and verbal exchanges between patients, doctors, providers, administrators, and other such stakeholders is often overlooked. (p. 7)

We—the researchers, theorists, scholars, and instructors in this field—are challenged to consider stakeholders' discourses that we previously might not have considered.

One study that accomplishes this is Bellwoar's (2012) case study, which is part of a larger study in which the researcher interviews user-patients who identify documents that influenced their health decisions. The project focuses on how users network and how "patients take up and remake medical discourse in their everyday lives for their own purposes" (p. 329). For the case study, Bellwoar follows Meagan, who was pregnant with complications and who used "texts to understand her body's functions, to manage her pain, and to develop relationships both personal with her baby and professional with her physicians" (Bellwoar, 2012, pp. 327–28). The study focuses on how Meagan used technical information, mingling genres and networks to be "actively literate" and to gather and analyze the data she might need to make informed decisions about her and her baby's health and well-being. Meagan did receive prenatal care during the study and consumed technical documents created and provided by physicians; however, she also "sought sources to make her own world" (Bellwoar, 2012, p. 331), asking friends for advice and resources, depending on her spouse's notes, and using alternative medicine to help with her ulcerative colitis. Meagan studied anatomical charts, listened to her own body, and responded to her body's messages:

> Finally, Meagan began to pinpoint the location of her pain precisely and use technical terms to describe it: "I'm feeling pain in my transverse colon." In this way, Meagan became an active participant in her diagnosis by integrating her previous knowledge and current research with the technical language that the physician needed to provide Meagan with adequate treatment. She positioned herself as a valid participant in her diagnosis because she alone was qualified to identify the location of her pain and articulate its quality to the doctors. Key to this articulation was the laminated nature of Meagan's literate activity—that is, the way her experiences as an artist, writer, and researcher came to be tied into her trajectory of literate action in identifying and articulating her pain. (Bellwoar, 2012, p. 338)

In this way, Meagan directed the communication that she gathered and analyzed and thus managed her own health and medical case. And in this study, Bellwoar (2012) illustrates how a patient makes new information by networking together the contents of cultural artifacts, visual documents, literate practices, and various media "to navigate future medical encounters" (p. 342). Bellwoar (2012) suggests that other researchers reimagine the scope of communication to literacies outside healthcare as well as to tests that "undo the privileging of patriarchal institutional spaces" (p. 343). In this study, the researcher also values and privileges the role of the patient to suggest "that technical communication researchers approach literate activity from the perspective of users' intentions and motives for technology use in their own worlds" (Bellwoar, 2012, p. 342). Her study illustrates the importance of a user's chain of multi-modal sources to synthesize information outside the traditional medical realm.

In her report *Living Chronic: Agency and Expertise in the Rhetoric of Diabetes*, Arduser (2017) also elevates patient voices. She shares that medical professions define *patient agency* as "the actions a patient takes outside of the clinical encounter to control blood sugar levels" (p. 2), and thus privilege the informed patient:

> According to medical and health care professionals, once a patient has received the necessary information, the person becomes an expert patient and possesses agency. The term *expert patient* . . . was coined by the United Kingdom's Department of Health following an observation made by doctors, nurses, and other health professionals that people with particular chronic diseases understand their disease better than a medical professional does. (p. 2)

By focusing on agency, Arduser (2017) establishes that individuals with diabetes are not receiving care but rather are "doing work," a distinction that justifies the voice of the patient because technical communication and the rhetorics of health and medicine both apply theories that relate to agency (p. 7) and thus task completion. Arduser (2017) openly states the strategy of her study: "putting the voices of diabetics and medical providers into conversation with each other . . . to honor voices by keeping them audible throughout the text. . . . In this case these discourses are those of lived experience and clinical medical knowledge" (p. 24). The voices she shares are in medical offices but are also present in online patient communities where patients discourse about diabetes:

> Here, the call and response may be the back and forth that goes on in a discussion thread online. Rather than agency being defined by the relationship between a writer and her text or a speaker and a listening audience, these interactions can be agential by virtue of the articulations between the people *in the room*, whether that is a physical or virtual meeting place. (Arduser, 2017, p. 74)

She expands this idea to explain that patients must do more than bring their experiences to their meetings with their healthcare providers; they must "develop a professional voice in these encounters" and thus learn from others and bring information, knowing what they are going to discuss in their appointments (Arduser, 2017, p. 147). She affirms that they can understand their diagnoses from interacting with other patients and thus can produce and share medical knowledge.[2]

Arduser's research lays a groundwork for researchers, theorists, advocates, and practitioners to further expand rhetoric by dignifying the voices of patient and patient experiences (without direct dependence on healthcare-provider involvement) to an elevated status within the medical and communication communities as valuable rhetorics of health and medicine. Patient voices, including patient discourse in online spaces, reflect the experience and research of those who, in addition to investigating and gathering information about their diseases, are living *through* disease and the disease process.

As stated earlier, traditionally, discussions of rhetorics of health and medicine related to the communication and persuasion of physicians with their colleagues, patients, and other healthcare providers. In this model, then, most frequently, providers are the rhetors, and patients and their families and advocates are the audiences; thus, the rhetorics of health and medicine began (before established as a field of its own) with a focus on the traditional medical community, defined as "the body of individuals who are qualified to practice medicine" (medical community, n.d.). Even as recent as 2009, critics state that the focus of medical discourse is physician-to-patient communication: "Unfortunately, much of the literature on medical discourse confines itself to practitioner-patient interaction in biomedical settings and tailors proposals for improving communication to biomedical models of the doctor-patient encounter" (Wilce, 2009, p. 201). As medicine shifts from a paternalistic model—with physicians making decisions and patients complying—to a partnership between practitioners and patients, the medical community and boundaries for the rhetorics of health and medicine are expanding to recognize the interdisciplinary focus of these communications (Angeli and Johnson-Sheehan, 2017; Scott, Segal, and Keränen, 2013), and scholars are illustrating the importance of including narratives created by patients—with their providers but also with each other. This scholarship "initiates inquiry into the role of rhetoric in various health care and medical discourses and examines what rhetoric—a discipline in its own right—can contribute to this . . . field" (Heifferon and Brown, 2000, p. 2). Therefore, scholars are establishing value for patient narratives in health and medical rhetorics. This expansion allows theorists to privilege patients and to allow patient voices to surface as equals within medical environments. That is, "the patient takes on certain new characteristics when regarded as a speaker and an audience involved in a rhetorical situation" (Segal, 2005, p. 37).

THIS STUDY OF PATIENT DISCOURSE

Researchers, theorists, and scholars in the rhetorics of health and science continue to call for more field-specific research (e.g., Angeli and Johnson-Sheehan, 2017; de Jong, 2009; Haas, 2009; Haswell, 2005; Hayhoe, 2006; Lang, 2009; McKee and Porter, 2008; *Present Tense* Editors, 2012; White-Farnham, Finer, and Molloy, 2017), as well as for more interdisciplinary and cultural research (e.g., Barton, 2001; Hayhoe, 2006; Lang, 2009; Rude, 2012) and for better defined research methods (e.g., Blakeslee and Spilka, 2004; Meloncon and Frost, 2015; Wilce, 2009). In response to these calls, this study applies traditional methods to new media with topics that overlap medical specialties, rhetoric, communication, and information architecture.

Other than to respond to these calls for diverse research, why should we study (and continue to study) the discourse between patients, specifically women, who are confronting breast cancer? A few of the reasons address the audiences for this book. First, for those who study the rhetorics of health and medicine, we are expanding our understanding of patient discourse, particularly as it relates to their discourse in medically focused online communities and to the rhetoric of breast cancer. In this way, we expand analysis of shared disease narratives and further establish patient voices in our field and in the medical community, as those patients are rhetors in medical discourse. Second, research of this discourse helps technical communicators and communication architects—those who may invest in media design for patients and for communities or who may mine data to research behavioral patterns and create persona of individuals in various cultures—to design better media for those who engage in these virtual spaces and also to anticipate complications related to the collection of potentially sensitive and personal nature that individuals self-disclose. (Chapter 5 addresses current trends in big data and how the future might affect individuals who post information online.) Third, through this discourse, we can consider what patients communicate and believe about their disease, their healthcare providers, and the disease process including how it affects their lives. This information can help in the transfer of medical communication as well as healthcare providers' investment in relationships with patients, as they better know what patients may expect and need. "What communication design from a rhetorical perspective can offer healthcare is a focus on patient experience, which includes an empathic focus found through our methods" (Meloncon and Frost, 2015, p. 11). We also need to consider how our methods, data sets, and studies establish standards for future research. Fourth, this study continues the adaptation of research methods from the social sciences into the study of the rhetorics of health and medicine. Researchers then must use the methods to refine and adapt them to be appropriate for use in rhetoric and communication studies. Included in these methods is the challenge to adapt standards of institutional review boards (IRBs) to address communication-related and online research. Currently, most review boards and their standards do not delineate how to handle research related to the rhetorics of health and medicine (King, Bivens, Pumroy, Rauch, and Koerber, 2017) and even more the interaction in online communities. This study advances the discussion of how ethics review boards like IRBs need to consider their applications and their standards for the research of patient discourse. (Chapter 4 includes a discussion of the ethical decisions that researchers need to consider to ensure that their research and publications do not direct unanticipated and uninvited audiences to potentially sensitive patient discourse.) Fifth, this study also expands on the ethical considerations for those who study patient discourse in online communities. This reason is particularly important as the U.S. healthcare system shifts and struggles over patients' pre-existing conditions. Although those conditions may be recorded in a patient's medical record, additional information in online discourse, particularly in a community of patients who are sharing experiences, can create additional documentation that could affect patients' future employment, insurability, and healthcare. In this way, this study continues to build the argument to advocate for patient privacy, confidentiality, security, and respect for online discourse as personal narrative as patients self-disclose online and as corporations mine data from virtual spaces that include information protected by Health Insurance Portability and Accountability Act (HIPAA). Finally, this study provides hope for patients who are diagnosed with breast cancer and for their families and friends who may feel like the patients' voices are drowned in the disease-related information and the statistics related to their diagnoses. *Patient voices matter.*

This study is about care—care for women and patients, care about ethical research, care regarding language and discourse, and care about healthcare:

> Care is a great way to center and help contextualize what it is that we do, and the approach to care would be a distinctly humanistic enterprise, that is, in helping us understand the deeply human aspects of what it means to be a patient or care giver or any other person within the health care system and what those people experience in that system. . . . Connecting our work to care and empathy illustrates the importance of the rhetorics of health and medicine as key to understanding or to gaining insights into what it means to experience the healthcare system. (Meloncon and Frost, 2015, p. 10)

In addition, care allows researchers to gain insight into what it means to experience illness. This care allows us to focus on the voices of patients—and in this study, the voices of women who are confronting breast cancer.

To investigate the discourse of patients in an online community, I considered what other scholars were reporting, I asked a small pool of breast-cancer patients about their concerns, I visited other online communities, and I analyzed patient-to-patient discourse on Breastcancer.org.

Review Board Approval

I identified Breastcancer.org, the largest online community related to breast cancer, for my study before I began. I had previously participated as a member of Breastcancer.org—during my mother's treatment for breast cancer—and then, when I decided to research the community, I removed myself by not signing in as a registered guest before visiting the site to collect artifacts for my study. At that point, I gathered and then analyzed a full thread of posts ("Progesterone Cream") and spent time observing posts and taking ethnographic notes on the community's public discussion board. As I studied, I began to feel concern about the privacy and confidentiality for the women who were posting the discussion-board posts. Therefore, I decided to submit my work for review by the institutional review board (IRB) at my institution to ensure that my work and processes followed guidelines for ethical research.

IRBs focus on the ethical design and implementation of research on human subjects, such as in surveys, focus groups, experimental and clinical investigations, and interviews—when the researcher has direct contact with the study participants. Because I was not investigating and gathering data from human subjects but was studying already-existing artifacts in a public online community, I was not required to apply for IRB approval. However, I decided to apply for accountability. My decision to apply created some complications because my study focused on the investigation of culture and rhetoric via text-based artifacts (created by humans) that were already published on the Internet in a public, non-password-protected discussion board. The IRB application was designed to review methods for studies of human subjects and to ensure anonymity (when necessary), confidentiality, privacy, and protection for human subjects—elements that I wanted for the women who created the artifacts I was studying; therefore, the application asked questions that were not relevant to my research, such as questions related to informed consent and anonymity. For example, the IRB application asked the following questions:

- How will you recruit participants for your study?
- What is the research instrument that you will use to collect data from your study participants?
- What task(s) will the participants be requested to perform?
- (For archival research) From what records or specimens will you collect data?

- What provisions will you take to maintain the privacy of subjects and confidentiality of data?

Research of online texts that are gathered from public discussion boards do not align with research from recruited participants, and the creators of the archives typically sign their posts with a username that they have chosen, knowing that they are publishing in a public online space. Therefore, I struggled with many of these questions. (I am not the only investigator who has struggled with the IRB application and its specifications toward basic-science research of human subjects because I was researching health-related communication via social science methods. Details about my struggle and the struggles of some of my fellow investigators is available in *Health Communication* [King, Bivens, Pumroy, Rauch, and Koerber, 2017].) I completed National Institutes of Health (n.d.) Office of Extramural Research training to protect human research participants and then applied to my IRB for approval under an application with "exempt status"—i.e., I was not gathering informed consent to contact the creators of the posts and ask for permission and I was not asking human subjects any potentially sensitive questions. After the IRB approved my study, with retroactive approval of my ethnographic work and of my analysis of the first thread, I gathered two additional threads of posts to analyze and continued to study the culture, taking ethnographic notes and learning from what I observed.

Because online posts in public spaces are pre-existing documents, some investigators readily justify the observation of these texts without IRB approval, stating that the Internet readily provides research data (Whitty and Joinson, 2009; Young, 2001). These texts are available "because users choose to participate in public areas of chat rooms . . . [therefore] those users implicitly give consent to observation" (Young, 2001, para. 8). The users of Breastcancer.org are instructed (Breastcancer.org—Community Guidelines, 2016) that anyone may access the posts in community areas. Other investigators, however, emphasize that individuals post online expecting their writings to remain personal (Im, Chee, Lim, et al., 2007; McKee and Porter, 2009, p. 6; Orgad, 2006, p. 179; Owen, Bantum, and Galant, 2009; Whitty and Joinson, 2009), and researchers should be wary of how we use their posted texts. Thus, researchers have a responsibility to consider, not the "subjects" or archives that make up the data, but the creators of that data and to protect them.

I was not required or even expected to apply for IRB approval before analyzing my first thread of posts. However, as I began to study the community of Breastcancer.org, I began to shift my opinions about IRB approval for investigations of online texts because of the sensitive and potentially personal nature of some of the content in the posts I was reading. In some of the posts, community members post information that is legally protected by

HIPAA, an act established to protect patients from the disclosure of personal, sensitive, and identifying information (DHHS, 2003). (I will address HIPAA more in chapter 4.) I submitted an application for expedited review through my IRB because I was not requesting the following from human subjects: data from vulnerable or under-aged participants, data of a sensitive nature, blinded medical records, or data with identifiable information. The IRB approved my application with no concerns.

Research Methods

A variety of research methods are appropriate, effective, and established for the analysis of discourse in an online public discussion board. Quantitative methods like experimental research, surveys, and content and meta analyses will answer the questions "how much," "how frequently," or "to what extent." In contrast, qualitative methods (including ethnographic methods, interviews, unobtrusive observation, case study, and historic and other analyses) allow a researcher to note the "how" and "why" of online community and member interactions. For this study, I chose to use ethnographic methods—a virtual ethnography—and a rhetorical analysis. Before I began my study, I submitted my methods to and imitated systematic methods used by other researchers (per Hughes and Hayhoe, 2008; MacNealy, 1999; Radin, 2006; Still, 2008) to be accountable for how I applied the method and to be ethical in my research.

(Of course, to fully and responsibly design my study, I became familiar with what other scholars have published in the corpus of literature related to breast cancer and communication, patient discourse, online community, the rhetorics of health and medicine, and the methods I was considering. I used keywords related to patient discourse and interaction, online communities, and breast cancer as well as more general searches related to online communities related to health and medical diagnoses and bibliographies of those articles gathered in the search. I used PubMed, EBSCO, and a variety of broader search engines as well as Google Scholar to identify sources related to the project to identify more than five hundred articles and books related to this project. Those resources that relate directly to this project and that informed and inspired the study are cited.)

Virtual Ethnography

First, I conducted a virtual ethnography of online communities related to health and medicine to study how communities were structured and how the members of those communities interacted. I also observed the community of Breastcancer.org, focusing on the structure and guidelines of that community as well as the member interaction as posts reflected members' expression of their concerns, preferences, advice, sources, and experiences.

Ethnographic research is traditionally a social-science method that enables the researcher to immerse herself in a culture and experience that culture as it swirls around her. My first exposure to ethnography was Scott Clark's (1994) *Japan, a View from the Bath.* Clark's ethnography, a study of the cultural connections of the Japanese bath, addresses the Japanese tradition of bathing to eliminate spiritual and mental "dirt." The ethnography, a three-month study of Clark's visits to Japanese baths, gives a powerful insight into the culture through the researcher's eyes, which are focused on experiencing, observing, and documenting the cultural elements related to that environment. Ethnography centers around the culture within a chosen community. "Classically, an ethnographer is often thought of as going out into a chosen field site, undertaking research into the culture encountered there, and coming back to write about the experience" (Hine, 2005, p. 7). Ethnographers uses rhetorical devices to gather information about the culture which they are investigating (Creswell, 2009, p. 194). Those rhetorical devices may include a variety of elements as well as addressing persuasion and *kairos* (considering the timing of the communication within the observed moments of the culture) and the *logos*, *ethos*, and *pathos* involved in the communication. Ethnography is a flexible research method, as it allows the researcher to adapt as the culture changes or as the researcher discerns when investigating a previously unknown culture or population; however, it is not a purposeless method (Hine, 2009, p. 6). The study is an appropriate method when little is known about a culture. "Ethnography has a larger scope [than other methods, like a case study]. It looks at a larger group such as a community, a cultural unit, or an environment, and it [the study] usually extends over a longer period of time" (MacNealy, 1999, p. 214). The length of time allows the researcher to observe more than a particularly moment in time in the culture and thus can observe elements of the culture over time to note consistency of the observations.

Virtual ethnography is an adaptation of the traditional research method ethnography to virtual environments to study the cultural elements that can be observed in virtual space. This adapted method then allows the researcher to investigate the textual (and sometimes video and visual) interaction of individuals who engage in online spaces:

> Observation in online research involves watching text and images on a computer screen rather than watching people in offline settings. However, the technologically mediated environment still provides direct contact with the social world the ethnographer is studying, since participants in that setting communicate through online behavior. (Garcia, Standlee, Bechkoff, and Cui, 2009, p. 58)

Thus, the investigator "experiences" (Garcia, Standlee, Bechkoff, and Cui, 2009, p. 59) or observes the behaviors of individuals in online spaces and then documents how those individuals rhetorically interact through their discourse. Virtual ethnographers immerse themselves in the texts published by community members (per Hine, 2009, p. 6), observing how members behave and interact via discourse and noting how they express their agency (Creswell, 2009, p. 194). The culture being investigated exists within a "chosen field site" (Hine, 2005, p. 6) in a virtual space; the researcher goes "into" a virtual community and then "returns" to write about the experience. By definition, this virtual, or online, ethnography describes the spaces: "Disembodied persons people these places. Such facts are the fuel of the cyberpunk imagination. For the ethnographer they create a more mundane dilemma: there is no obvious place to 'go' to carry out fieldwork. Rather, data collection seems more a matter of deskwork" (Rutter and Smith, 2005, p. 84). The data is collected from within the online community, with the researcher never leaving her desk to travel (geographically and physically) to some foreign place. This research method allows for a shift and thus the collection of cultural artifacts *in situ*, which allows the investigator to maintain the integrity of the artifact's context.

Qualitative Analysis

Second, I conducted qualitative analysis on the artifacts for this study—I sampled the discourse in the community, collecting three publicly posted threads and then analyzing in three phases: observing the discourse, noting and coding observations, and analyzing those elements to identify themes and patterns (Hughes and Hayhoe, 2008, p. 78). Of course, the researcher should choose a proven method, because "if the methodology isn't sound, the conclusions and subsequent recommendations won't be sound" (Goubil-Gambrell, 1992, p. 583). I chose a sound method and maintained the integrity of the context of these posts so I could qualitatively analyze the posts with consideration of how they fit into the culture of this medically focused online community. A variety of qualitative methods and analyses per various communication theories are appropriate and established to study online discourse.

Discourse analysis is "analyzing text" (Hughes and Hayhoe, 2008, p. 23), and studying discourse expands our body of knowledge per the speaker and audience as well as the context for the discourse (MacNealy, 1999, p. 124). Rhetorical analysis is categorized as discourse analysis, which typically depends on the principle of categorization (MacNealy, 1999, p. 131); it allows the investigator to deconstruct members' communication, analyzing the community members rhetoric per the who, what, when, where, why, and how they are communicating. Discourse analyses, and specifically rhetorical analysis, pair well with ethnography, as both focus on the rhetorical elements: "To conduct a rhetorical analysis, then, is to conduct an analysis of the culture, of the discourse, that surrounds the words, the norms, the systems that shape, in this case, past medical practice . . . and a resulting alternative rhetoric that has served to modify perception and practice. . . . Rhetoric is representative of and contributor to a complex, dynamic discourse of values, truths, and rules" (Still, 2008, p. 2).

Aristotelian rhetorical analysis allows the researcher to consider the persuasive tones of the discourse, focusing on the speaker's *logos, ethos,* and *pathos* and how the speaker uses emotion and empathy, character and credibility, and logic to connect with and to influence the audience. Rhetorical analysis can also be framed by Burke's theory and method of Dramatism, which considers motive: "[A]ny complete statement about motives will offer some kind of answers to these five questions: what was done (act), when or where it was done (scene), who did it (agent), how he did it (agency), and why (purpose)" (Burke, 1969, p. xv). Various other frames (such as Bormann's Symbolic Convergence Theory and Fantasy Analysis and Fisher's Narrrative Paradigm Theory) can be used to research and analyze discourse. The method also depends on the focus the researcher is taking in analyzing the discourse: e.g., to analyze the rhetoric (persuasion), the narrative and the structure and social roles of stories, or the conversation and minute details of interaction.

Other researchers have analyzed online texts with other methods—through case studies, discourse and textual analyses, and general qualitative analysis—but most begin with limited categories. For example, Radin (2006) analyzed messages from Breast Cancer Action Nova Scotia (BCANS) and reported that BCANS "comprises 5 [*sic*] main thematic sections, or fields of emphasis: interactive messages, self-introduction, information, fundraising" (p. 598). She categorized messages in her study in four categories: support, queries, news and information, and projects (Radin, 2006, pp. 596–697). Similarly, Blank and Adams-Blodnieks (2007) analyzed the content of messages on two WebMD asynchronous bulletin boards: one for breast cancer and one for prostate cancer. These investigators identified "four main categories of content—medical/treatment, intimacy/sexuality, emotional expression, and support" (p. 1249) and later added two additional categories: economic and miscellaneous. They stated that they did not use uniform coding, even though they were aware of other researchers' codes, but instead allowed categories to emerge through Blank and Adams-Blodnieks' analysis of the text (2007, p. 1252). Their emphasis then was coding information within the posts rather than analyzing the actions or intents of the community members who created the posts.

Studies like these have too rigorously limited the analysis of messages from community members and have muted rich layers of information, agency, identity, and relationships that are evident through ethnographic study. "The limitation of most of the existing studies of these aspects is that they replicate findings across various patient-related online contexts. The claims they make are usually, general, hackneyed and obvious: that 'patients use the Internet to share information, express their feelings and offer support'" (Orgad, 2006, p. 16). Orgad argued for a more relaxed coding scheme, one in which investigators can allow the text to lead the researcher rather than the researcher forcing the text into previously and externally created categories. This relaxed coding method in qualitative analysis more consistently aligns with a "flexible and fluid" method (Hughes and Hayhoe, 2008) that is non-scripted (Jones, 1999a, p. xiii). This coding method does not deny the investigator's ability to consider and even use codes from previous analyses or research projects; however, it eliminates boundaries that might influence the investigator's ability to analyze the content without bias and thus allow more unique elements in the data to surface.

I eliminated my own scholarly bias and restrictions on data and observations in a variety of ways. My focus was to learn about the culture of the community and the members who were interacting online by analyzing their discourse—how they used language to connect and act. Therefore, imitating other studies, I chose three diverse threads—one from new members of the community, one from members with a specific diagnosis of breast cancer, and one from members who had been through most of their treatment and were discussing issues related to their care—to triangulate my findings. (By triangulating, I was able to look at very different posts and compare the discourse going on in different spaces in the same community. These threads of posts differed per size, time, membership represented, purpose, and tone. The members were in various stages of the disease process—just diagnosed, in treatment, and recovering—and addressed breast cancer in different ways, as I will discuss in chapters 2 and 3.) I also journaled and annotated as I moved through the text so I could identify unique, relevant, and thought-provoking elements in the discourse; this method is described by Farkas and Haas (2012) in their discussion of qualitative analysis methods and grounded theory, where they state that "writing [should become] a central strategy" (p. 13) from the very beginning of a qualitative analysis. Writing notes throughout the analysis process "allow[s] for the discovery of unexpected knowledge" (Hughes and Hayhoe, 2008, p. 8).

The common element of qualitative analysis is coding—the categorizing and subcategorizing of content to analyze the data—but the difference is the researcher's motive in coding: i.e., what is the researcher investigating. Coding is a challenging part of the process, although computer software has simplified the work. I began my analysis coding and recording on paper, with colored paper tabs on print copies of the data, and in Microsoft Excel, which provides a spreadsheet presentation of data—valuable for categorization. Chunks of discourse can be numbered by sentences, lines, paragraphs, posts, members, etc. However, Excel is limited in the dimension of documentation and is a more valuable tool for quantitative analysis; I found that I was unable to observe posts in context, an important part of my analysis. Therefore, I shifted to NVivo, which expanded my observations and allowed me to write notes as well as code, connecting my notes, observations, and diverse codes to the same data. NVivo allows the researcher to use an open-coding method and cluster codes into larger categories, called nodes, and then largest, most general categories, called trees (Hoover and Koerber, 2011, p. 4; QSR International, 2010). Researchers can also use tags in the texts (Remler and Van Ryzin, 2011) to create variables, codes, or "constructs of interest" (MacNealy, 1999). ("One of the keys to strong qualitative analysis is effective management of vast arrays of data" [Hoover and Koerber, 2011, p. 4].) My codes were defined by the content of the text, although I did have prior knowledge from observations from my virtual ethnography and relevant studies from my literature review (Anderson and Klemm, 2008; Beaudoin and Tao, 2007; Bradley, 2008; Bunde, Suis, Martin, and Barnett, 2006; Dickerson, Boemhmke, Ogle, and Brown, 2006; Im, Chee, Lim, Lui, Guevara, and Kim, 2007; Lieberman and Goldstein, 2006). Coding is a complex process; "researchers seldom proceed in simple linear fashion through this . . . sequence" (Huckin, 2004, p. 16). Coding is also a reiterative process; the researcher must consider the content and document codes until obvious categories and themes emerges. With NVivo, the researcher can conduct a "broad brush analysis" or automatic coding (QSR International, 2010) to automatically capture words and synonyms that fit within the same code. Coding should be conducted in small, complete chunks of text in each sitting with notes and annotated memos to explain the researcher's observations (Bazeley, 2007; Farkas and Haas, 2012).

Coding can continue to a point of saturation: "[when] no additional data are being found whereby the sociologist can develop properties of the category. As he sees similar instances over and over again, the researcher becomes empirically confident that a category is saturated" (Glaser and Strauss, 1999, p. 61). Saturation is also "the point at which staying another day, interviewing another respondent, or testing another user ceases to add any new data. . . . [Y]ou would not know where data saturation occurs until . . . you start observing the same themes or behaviors occurring with no new insight or data being added" (Hughes and Hayhoe, 2005, p. 81). At that point, data collection becomes redundant in the sample. When codes begin to seem redundant, the researcher should re-evaluate codes, establish new units, and repeat the process until coding is complete.

In my analysis, I created 222 nodes from three threads and 676 posts from 124 unique members of the community present on the public discussion board of Breastcancer.org. The quantification of the posts and codes does not equate to conclusions in a qualitative analysis; however, I did note patterns in community members' participation—that is, some members were more active in threads than others were. I note that frequency in my analysis (in chapters 3 and 4) to identify the activity of members in the community. (Breastcancer.org also notes how many posts members have posted to identify those who are newcomers, those who infrequently post, and those who are actively discoursing in the online space.) I also built on my coding schemes; in other words, when I created a code in the first analysis, I maintained that code in the coding scheme for use in the other two threads, and I returned to threads to analyze new codes until I truly reached saturation. For complex information, I coded content but also recorded annotations and memos in NVivo (Bazeley, 2007; Durian, 2002, p. 739; Farkas and Haas, 2012); those notes have been inserted in appropriate places throughout my analysis reporting.

Issues with Methods

In my sample selection and coding, I faced two particular issues. First, I wanted to ensure the rigor and replicability of the study I was conducting, and second, I wanted to focus on women's voices in the posts that I was analyzing.

My first concern was that "[healthcare research] shares a concern about rigor and lack of generalizability that is evident in some of our field's major research. . . . [Q]ualitative research that does not provide adequate description of sampling techniques renders questionable interpretation and replication of that research" (Koerber and McMichael, 2008, p. 461). Another researcher expressed a similar concern: "Because there is no randomization of subjects, no identification of variables, and no treatment it is important that the qualitative researcher provide readers with a full description of the setting where . . . and how they were collected" (Goubil-Gambrell, 1992, p. 588). Concerns that studies are not rigorous or replicable and cannot be generalized are valid because unique studies that do little for our field's body of research also do little to adapt and establish research methods. To address these concerns, I submitted my methods to other researchers before I began my study and, in my methods, imitated other studies (e.g., Blank and Adams-Blodnieks, 2007; Still, 2008). I also replicated my own study three times on three separate threads of posts to refine my methods so that other researchers can apply the same methods and theories to future studies to better understand discourse in other online communities. By imitating established studies, by submitting my design with documented methods to other investigators and to my IRB, and by conducting my research on three separate threads of posts in separate analyses, I addressed this first concern.

Second, I searched for any gender-specific references in the threads—any references to being male—so I could focus my analysis on females' posts. I did not investigate the community members outside the posts I was analyzing: i.e., I did not use the usernames related to or the identifying information within the posts to learn more about the community members (including to learn about their gender). Some of the posts were easy to filter: for example, the thread called "Progesterone Cream" is a collection of posts from women who are discussing hormone-replacement therapy—medicinal and homeopathic—because of deficiency resulting from or after treatment for breast cancer. Males can experience progesterone deficiency, as progesterone is a hormone in men's and women's systems (Oettel and Mukhopadhyay, 2004), so men could participate in the discourse focused on progesterone cream; however, I did not note any references to male progesterone deficiency or any references from the members writing posts about being male. I included all posts in the three threads because none of the community members specified that they were male; however, numerous posts indicated that the writers were female. (I will address some of those posts in chapters 3 and 4.) In this way, I addressed my second concern, including all posts in the three threads because none of the posts included male-specific comments.

I do not exclude male voices to silence those voices or to indicate that male voices related to breast cancer are not relevant; males are diagnosed with breast cancer (less than 1 percent of cases; National Breast Cancer Foundation, Inc., 2016) and through the experiences of their loved ones. I focus on women's voices to prioritize those because they are predominant in discourse related to breast cancer and because I chose to focus on women's voices for this study. (Breastcancer.org does have threads that are male specific, and male voices are a small part of the rhetoric of breast cancer. Future research should include those few male voices and should focus on differences between male and female voices and their rhetorics as they relate to breast cancer.)

Research Data

Certain terms are relevant to the data that are gathered from online discourse that is published in a public discussion board; online discourse is organized differently than are other media and content. Online discourse (text-based content published as hypertext) is considered an artifact—an already established text that has been published in an online space—and the content is organized in *posts* that are categorized in *threads*. A post has only one author and is published at a set time within the discussion board. Each post contains a subject, a date/time stamp, and a signature from the author. The initial post (a posted question or prompt) in a conversation starts a thread: a string of posts that ideally are related to one topic and are conversations of responses to previous posts. Once a member has posted the initial post, other members can reply, building the length and the content and richness of the thread. As a result, the initial post defines the focus for that thread. On the discussion board, the posts in a thread are typically posted in the reverse chronological order of their publishing.

The conversation within a thread is not live or synchronous; individuals may be online at the same time but will not be publishing at the same time or immediately responding, as they do in face-to-face discourse. Thus, the conversation may be built over time with asynchronous text-based posts; it is not limited by the members' availability at any one time but instead allows them to participate in the conversation and respond when convenient to previous posts in the thread.

A thread is typically titled so members of the online community know the initial focus of discourse. A thread is a conversation but it is also a construct of organization of discourse: posts are published in the order in which they are submitted. These constructs together are data that illustrate and support cultural practices within the community. Posts and threads are called *artifacts*—hypertext that exists at one point in time and thus is a snapshot of a discussion board. The communication within artifacts is not live, but the content is organic and may change at any time when another post or thread is added to the online artifact.

Individuals who post artifacts are called *members* and, within Breastcancer.org, they are individuals who have registered to interact within the online community. Members may or may not participate. What differentiates members from visitors to the online community is that they are registered, even with only a username, and thus can post in the online community. Currently, Breastcancer.org has 183,000 members and 139,000 threads; the corpus of text in this online archive is too large for a study and also is alive, constantly growing as individuals join and as members post. Other communities also are open for large numbers of members—membership is not limited to geographic proximity and thus is open to anyone who has access to the Internet and the community pages.

For this study, I could not study a full collection of the threads of artifacts available via Breastcancer.org; therefore, I chose a sample of threads at different times via a purposeful sampling method with consistent criteria for the artifacts, as other researchers have done (e.g., Koerber and McMichael, 2008, p. 465). This purposeful sampling allows for a diverse sample: the members are registered with Breastcancer.org and have been diagnosed (or were representing a family member who has been diagnosed), but the threads differ in content because the members are in different stages of the disease process—diagnosis, treatment, and recovery—and thus in their experiences with breast cancer. The threads also differ in format, length, intent, and member characteristics. These differences enhance the findings of the study by providing members who have different perspectives, resources, questions, and purposes and by allowing the observation of a broader scope of topics with information-rich posts (per Goubil-Gambrell, 1992, p. 588). The data represent a larger sample of posts on the discussion board (per Koerber and McMichael, 2008, p. 464), which is vital for generalizable research.

I thoughtfully chose three threads of posts as the data set for this study:

- "Progesterone Cream" includes 469 posts (within 4 months, 2 days) from women who have finished or soon will finish their treatments for breast cancer and are interacting to discourse about medicinal and homeopathic progesterone treatment and related issues;
- "MPBC" includes 31 posts (within 12 days) from women who have been diagnosed with metaplastic breast cancer, a rare form of breast cancer, and who communicate to discuss that particular diagnosis; and
- "Just Diagnosed" includes 176 posts (within 10 months) from women who recently have received their diagnoses of breast cancer and from women who previously were diagnosed and communicate in this thread to help newly diagnosed community members.

The diversity of these threads allowed me to analyze discourse and narratives from a diverse pool of women; their discussions differ in stage of cancer, stage of life, lifestyle, values, locations, type and stage of cancer, and a variety of other characteristics. And, by choosing three diverse threads that contained 676 posts from 124 unique members of the community, I seek to address the entire population of the community.

OUTLINE OF CHAPTERS

This book contains five chapters. Chapter 1 addresses online communities and the patient discourse that occurs in medically focused communities—specifically Breastcancer.org. The chapter includes the traditional definitions of *community* and *discourse* and then addresses how these terms apply to virtual versions of the concepts. Chapter 2 addresses the rhetoric of breast cancer, starting with the tradition of rhetoric and then shifting to address how the community of individuals who are affected by breast cancer have its own rhetoric and uses it within the community to discourse, advocate, and strengthen that community. Chapter 3 focuses on patients and how they communicate about medical care in this online community. These patients seek to express their agency in their own medical care, sharing their experiences—positive and negative—with their healthcare providers, pharmaceutical companies, and other members of the medical community. This chapter also addresses the struggle in medical care between basic sciences and alternative and complementary medicine from the perspective of the patients. Chapter 4 shifts to ethical and legal considerations that an online researcher must face, that relate to patient privacy and security, and that patients disclose online. This chapter also includes a discussion about the ethical challenges of quoting online discourse without traditional citations—to alleviate the possibility that unintended audiences will interrupt the community or visit and influence particularly sensitive posts on Breastcancer.org. Finally, chapter 5 begins a conversation on the future of patient discourse per big data and how corporations are mining information from the Internet. This chapter is relevant and poses challenges for the future of online communities because many patients are posting HIPAA-protected information in public (non-password-protected) discussion boards and communities, information that is readily available and gathered for analysis.

FUTURE RESEARCH

This book presents the results of four years of research; however, the findings also suggest even more questions than those that fueled the project. These questions relate to the diversity of the community around women diagnosed with breast cancer—the diversity of their diseases and the related disease processes, the variety of perspectives as they relate to culture and ethnicity, and the needs that different women need around the globe and how those needs relate to the rhetoric of breast cancer.

Breast cancer is category of diseases. "The term 'breast cancer' refers to a malignant tumor that has developed from cells in the breast" ("What is breast cancer?" 2017, para. 3). Different breast cancers develop from the mutation of different cells throughout the breast; different cancers include ductal carcinoma *in situ*, various types of invasive ductal carcinoma, invasive lobular carcinoma, inflammatory breast cancer, and metastatic breast cancer. The cancer is labeled by where the mutation begins and is staged by the size of tumor. The patient's diagnosis also considers how far the cancer has spread: that is, are the cancerous cells contained within the tumor, have they entered into the patient's blood stream (as evident by their presence in the lymph nodes), or have they spread and developed tumors in other parts of the patient's system (body). Therefore, patients who are diagnosed with breast cancer experience diverse specific diagnoses, treatments, recovery processes, and outcomes.

Breastcancer.org is a resource with a community started by a U.S. breast surgeon via a U.S.-based URL. Although this community's members are identified mostly as patients in the United States—members usually provide their location in their signature and profile and sometimes in their discourse—some members identify themselves as residents of France, Australia, and the United Kingdom. Regardless of their geographic location, they do open the discussion of patient discourse beyond one medical facility to allow for the boundary-less existence of online networks and the potential for "global citizenry" (Scott, Segal, and Keränen, 2013, p. 2) as it relates to the rhetoric of breast cancer. Their experiences with the disease process and healthcare differ per their location. Future research may identify how patients going through the disease process in different locations are experiencing different care and communicate these differences.

In the same way, patients from different ethnicities and cultures will have different experiences with breast cancer. Breast cancer is a global concern (Coughlin and Ekwueme, 2009) and is becoming a greater and more public issue, particularly in South Eastern Asia and Arab countries. Medical and epidemiologic research shows that, unlike the United States where breast cancer incidence is decreasing (or at least plateauing; Ravdin, Cronin, Howlader, et al., 2007), the incidence of breast cancer in Asia is increasing, and some South East Asian groups are experiencing lower survival rates after breast-cancer diagnosis (Bhoo-Pathy, Hartman, Saxena, et al., 2012). Breast cancer rates in Eastern Asia are estimated to have risen in last decade: 30 percent in China and India and as much as 100–200 percent in Japan, Korea, and Singapore (Bhoo-Pathy, Hartman, Saxena, et al., 2012). Breast cancer rates are rising quickly in Arab populations (e.g., North Africa and the Middle East) as well (Chouchane, Boussen, and Sastry, 2013). Therefore, future research needs to consider how patients from different backgrounds and cultures discourse about breast cancer.

Future research may also focus on the rhetoric of breast cancer within a male population: to investigate if male patients use the same persuasion, the same rhetorical devices, and the same appeals that female patients use. Men are experienced with breast cancer. Their experiences are different because they are facing a disease that most of society connects with women (even with the color pink) and they do not experience the loss of an identity-connected organ. Other male-specific experiences, needs, and emotions may be relevant. Future research should investigate the rhetorical practices of male patients.

This book responds to the call for expanded knowledge and statues of rhetoric within different communities and patient populations. Patients have diverse health and medical needs and experiences; some are seeking community centered around health and medical needs related to pregnancy, lactose intolerance, breast feeding, other cancers, kidney failure, depression, diabetes, obesity. Many patients are gathering in online communities to discuss their needs, diagnoses, and treatments and to create relationships with others who are experiencing the same health or medical circumstances. Their diseases bring unique experiences and rhetoric that relates to the specific diagnosis and their voices bring value to the rhetorics of health and medicine. Future research needs to investigate these rhetorics: "communication about health and medicine is ever more important in shaping our understandings of our cultures, our politics, and ourselves" (Meloncon and Frost, 2015, p. 8), and future research should continue to include patient voices "to access a broader spectrum of participant perspectives" (by Scott, Segal, and Keränen, 2013, p. 3).

NOTES

1. My mother's experiences are shared with her permission.
2. Arduser (2017) notes that a subset of patients are informed and experienced enough about their chronic illness to be considered expert patients. Some critics disagree with the term "expert" for patients, as Kopelson (2009) and Owens (2011) discuss in their articles.

Chapter One

Online Communities and Patient Discourse

People are drawn to others who are like them (Hart, Albarracin, Eagly, Brechan, Lindberg, and Merrill, 2009). These clusters of people, as they grow, build stronger relationships and develop into communities. The word *community* comes from the Latin words *com* and *unus*; *com* means "with" or "together," and *unus* means "singularity" or represents the number one (Harper, 2016). Community brings together singular units (Delanty, 2009, p. x) to create a focused group:

> a unified body of individuals, as . . . people with common interests living in a particular area . . . ; a group of people with a common characteristic or interest living together within a larger society; a group linked by common policy; a body of persons or nations having a common history or common social, economic, and political interests. (Community, 2012)

These common characteristics can include demographics like gender, socioeconomic level, or age; (dis)ability; medical diagnosis or need; background (such as the members' culture, education, ethnicity, or family structure); values (like religious or political preference, lifestyle, or priorities); and experiences (such as profession, training, skills, interests, or activities). "Community have been based on ethnicity, religion, class or politics; they may be large or small; 'thin' or 'thick' attachments may underlie them; they may be locally based or globally organized; they may be affirmative or subversive in their relation to the established order; they may be traditional, modern or even postmodern; they may be reactionary or progressive" (Delanty, 2010, p. xi). In communities, members gather because of some evident commonality or interest.

TRADITIONAL COMMUNITY

The definition of community may be influenced by the field in which the theorist works (Hamman, 1997); psychology, sociology, anthropology, communication, engineering, medicine, and other fields have their own definitions. For example, a government document focuses on the characteristics of those involved and the actions of the group, using policy terms to define community: "a relatively homogenous human population, within a defined area, experiencing little mobility, interacting and participating in a wide range of local affairs, and sharing an awareness of common life and personal bonds" (Dalton and Dalton, 1975, as cited in Walmsley, 2000, p. 5). Sociology-focused definitions propose more than ninety characteristics of a community (Hamman, 1997; Reich, 2010) or allow for a broad definition of people involved and simplifies these characteristics to define community with general terms: "(1) a group of people (2) who share social interaction (3) and some common ties between themselves and the other members of the group (4) and who share an area for at least some of the time" (Hamman, 1997, para. 4). A psychiatrist's definition focuses on eight actions of a community to define the characteristics of those within the group, stating that members

- accept and commit to each other, making decisions democratically;
- bring diverse perspectives;
- consider their relationship with the world;
- are transparent and can share vulnerability;
- experiment with peacemaking and appreciation for others;
- disagree, but with grace;
- share in leadership and work together; and
- share in the spirit of the community—"peace, love, wisdom, and power" (Peck, 1987, as cited by economist McKay, 2010, p. 26).

An anthropologist's definition focuses on "a performance—something that a group accomplishes together and before one another within a subjective and material context" (Goodsell and Williams, 2008, p. 253); this definition focuses on what the group can do through action together. A geographer's definition also considers action, focusing on "interaction not place that is the essence of urban life" (Walmsley, 2000, p. 6), although a shared physical location is necessary in this description of community. In a medically focused study, participants define a community as having five elements—"locus, sharing, joint action, social ties, and diversity" (MacQueen, McLellan, Metzer, et al., 2001, p. 1930), whereas the investigators define community as "a group of people with diverse characteristics who are linked by social ties, share common perspectives, and engage in joint action in geographical locations or settings" (MacQueen, McLellan, Metzer, et al., 2001, p. 1929). Other definitions may focus on what members accomplish or choose as interests or goals but also consider who is in the community and how they gather and discuss or accomplish these shared goals.

An inclusive definition with a multidisciplinary tone shares three common elements to describe a community. Social scientist Walmsley (2000) generalizes to say that all communities have "a geographic area," "a local social system centered around interaction between people and institutions," and "a human association founded on personal ties and a sense of belonging ([referencing] Urry, 1995)" (p. 5). These definitions establish foundations for the shared characteristics of a community.

Communities should be identified per qualitative evaluation—per their characteristics and the benefits that they bring to the humans who make up the membership. Slanina and Konopasek (2010) published empirical research with a quantitative method to evaluate an online group to determine if that group was a community. They report, "We want to introduce and illustrate a new mathematical method for identification of small parts of complex networks with higher levels of commonalities for studying their basic formal properties" (Slanina and Konopasek, 2010, p. 700). However, communities rarely can be evaluated quantitatively through stereotypes and inflexible standards that limit human interaction. If researchers consider qualitative data—such as how many active participants are in the group, how often these members participate, how quickly their membership grows, how many objectives the members together accomplish, and what language the membership shares and uses—we can quantify membership and interaction. However, this method does not allow for the qualities— the "sense of belonging" or "personal ties" that define community (e.g., Walmsley, 2000)—of a community and of the relationships between members. This sense of belonging and interpersonal elements are identified through qualitative and interpretive assessment; that is, community must be defined and described by the structure of the community as well as the shared purpose of the membership and the interactions of the members.

Researchers sometimes also use the term *community* in their analyses to describe the groups they are studying (e.g., Anwar, Chae, Natriello, 2010; Byrn, 2008; Suler, 2004; Zaugg, West, Tateishi, and Randall, 2011) rather than to define what a community is. Those who do define community and use the term for a group of people typically are focusing on the particular group which they are investigating. However, community is more than one group; community needs to be generalized to allow for diverse characteristics that allow for the preferences and perspectives of the members. As a result, the definition of *community* and the characteristics of a community are vital to shifting that definition to include groups that fit into the definition and bear those characteristics but do so using recently developed tools together. Three common characteristics allow for a focus on the membership; those characteristics are shared purpose, structured environment, and interaction and relationship.

Shared Purpose

Community members gather because they share a purpose, an interest, or a characteristic. Various theories and definitions of community exist around the members' shared purpose, which other theorists identify as "common interests, motives, ideas, or objectives" (Kotowski and dos Santos, 2010, p. 151; see also Cassidy, 2011; Huffaker, 2010; Nah, 2010; Wenger, 2006). The members may live in the same neighborhood; practice the same faith; enjoy the same game; support the same political agenda or candidate; live similar lifestyles; or share characteristics such as demographics, education, lifestyle, needs, or medical diagnoses. These groups gather to act with that shared purpose, such as to discuss an opinion and make decisions about the public area of their neighborhood, to worship corporately and merge their resources to share their purpose, to play together, to discuss challenges, to cheer for their alma mater, or to inspire and market their opinions to the public. Through that shared purpose, members adapt to the community culture—the language, the membership, the expectations, and the behaviors.

The purpose that members share may be as simple as their desire to belong, something that all humans seek (Gangadharbatla, 2008). "No man is an island, entire of himself; every man is a piece of the continent, a piece of the main" (Donne, 1999, p. 103), and "It is not good for man to be alone" (Genesis 2:18, Douay-Rheims Version). Human beings need each other and need relationship. They may share an interest or purpose, but the desire to belong to a group is a basic motivator that may encourage and drive members to belong and thus invest in the community. It has social value:

> The concept of community in classical sociology and community studies has been challenged by developments relating to cosmopolitanism, postmodernism, globalization, migration and the Internet. Far from disappearing, as the classical sociologists believed, community as a contemporary resonance in the current social and political situation, which appears to have produced a worldwide search for roots, identity and aspirations for belonging. (Delanty, 2010, p. x)

Modern society is unpredictable; individuals are no longer limited in the individuals they can find and in the relationships they can create. Relationships are changing as technology is expanding the who, what, when, where, why, and how of interaction—through technology such as the telegraph and then the telephone, the computer, the mobile phone, and the Internet. Yet, the "sufficient human feeling" (Rheingold, 1993) of belonging creates a bond between members.

Structured Environment

A community exists in a structured environment: in a location with membership standards, expectations, and/or requirements and with governance. Location for a traditional community is a physical space where the community meets: perhaps a meeting room, a restaurant, a neighborhood, a place of worship, an office, or another place that will physically house the members of the community. But environment is not limited to geography, which allows online groups that gather for a purpose and interact together to also be categorized as communities.

More influential to community members than the geographic location is the structure of the group's environment, and structure centers around membership standards. Communities establish requirements for membership—such as members must live in a particular community, practice a certain faith, graduate from a particular school, or even simply choose to be a member of the community (acting on their desire to belong). These requirements may be established before the community begins to develop or they may develop as the community grows. They may be determined by community members or they may be established by administrators or founders, or the decisions can be shared. These requirements determine the *who* of membership and also connect with what members must do to be members of the community: they may need to apply for membership, pay an annual membership fee, or attend a certain number of gatherings. They may also be required to follow membership standards to determine their behavior as members.

The governance of the community may be the administrators who create the organization, the elected leadership, or employed governance that enforces the membership requirements and standards. The governance exists to specify membership and also to ensure the safety and rights of those who exist and participate within the community. For example, you may be a member of the homeowners' association, but you must live in a specific neighborhood and pay a regular fee to invest in the community, and you must follow a set of rules lest the association management send you warning letters and then put a lien on your property. The same is true for an online community, because you may be required to register and abide by certain guidelines that outline what is acceptable online behavior. These elements for members may be as complicated and costly as a country-club membership or may be as simple and undemanding as being part of a fan club or a group of people who meet monthly (or when they can) to play a game.

Interaction and Relationship

Most characteristic of a community is the bond between members that connects and draws them together—the interaction and relationship between the members. This interaction is the characteristic that distinguishes a community from the public. Without relationship, people have no communal interest in the shared purpose, which eliminates the accountability of the structure of the community. But with interaction and relationships, community members build personal conscience that encourages them to invest in the best of others or at least in the shared purpose. Thus, in communities, individuals act and interact with others (Chou, Min, Change, and Lin, 2010; Iriberri and Lery, 2009; Reich, 2010; Wenger, 2006) as they converse, call each other by name, and reference previous interactions and conversation chains to build and maintain discourse. As members converse, they solidify their commitment to the space, their emotional involvement, and their sense of belonging to members within that group.

Community requires some sense of commitment, as noted in the previous section about registration, and a commitment to a shared purpose. Thus, these three characteristics of community cannot be separated. But interaction is vital to the existence of a community; a group without interaction is just a group and cannot be categorized as a community. The question arises if those who visit the community—the person who silently attends the homeowners' association meeting or sits in the back of the class and does not interact with the other students—is part of the community. That person may be a member, but without interaction and relationship with other members, through speaking with others or consistently attending meetings and recognizing other members, that individual does not invest to build a community. A community thrives when the members relate and interact.

ONLINE COMMUNITY

People communicate about shared interests—products, services, entertainment, health, hobbies, interests, priorities, and even medical diagnoses. As they interact, they develop relationships, and as relationships develop, so do communities. And people are finding community online: they are searching the Internet via a search engine to apply keywords related to their interests and goals and then joining online groups that center around those keywords and goals. They create face-to-face communities, but they also create and establish online communities that extend beyond traditional boundaries; technology is eliminating those boundaries. Technology allows individuals to seek community in new ways, motivated by their desire to belong (Gangadharbatla, 2008, p. 8). With technology—man-made machines—we can "gather news from the other side of the world or from family and friends nearby through digital social networks . . . [to] convey your thoughts or make requests to people almost anywhere on the globe" (Ryan, 2015, p. 1). As technology becomes more and more a tool for interaction and communication, people are changing the way they meet and interact to use tools that eliminate the element of distance and geography (and also limit the element of time), and they are creating community online via social media, instant messaging, and online forums. They are making friends online. They are locating missing family members. They are finding dates and love. They are advocating online, participating in causes by donating money, asking questions, gathering information, and sharing facts and stories about issues and events. They are attending school via the Internet, studying online sources and interacting with classmates in online spaces and virtual classrooms. They are participating in political, religious, and policy debates through their online connections, surrounding themselves with followers, acquaintances, and friends with whom they converse and share information. Technology is allowing individuals to classify the people with whom they interact so they can cluster in online spaces with those who have something in common with them. In other words, the Internet is allowing individuals to create online communities. The development of online community has no boundaries and is exciting.

As researchers and rhetoricians adapt traditional rhetorical theories to apply to communication via new media and in new rhetorical situations, they must also adapt traditional research methods to investigate new content, media, and audiences. Traditional methods from the social sciences allow communication researchers to systematically gather data from samples of texts, participants, and other data sets to analyze how people interact; these traditional methods can include surveying; case studies; observation; field research; focus groups; and qualitative and quantitative analyses such as content, rhetorical, discourse, and textual analyses. Methods depend on what the researcher expects to investigate and, because the research seeks to investigate large populations, the researcher must systematically isolate a sample that can be assessed.

Theorists and researchers continue to argue whether the definition of *community* can be expanded (Bell, 2001) to include online communities. As the world becomes more Internet-centric and the global environment becomes commonplace, theorists need a global definition that merges already-accepted definitions for traditional community and allows for a multidisciplinary perspective to delineate what an online community is. The previously accepted definitions for *online community* (and several are cited earlier in this chapter) are inadequate because they are static; they limit people as society and communication change and define community around the *where* and *how* rather than around the *who* and *what*. In particular, the definitions create controversy between a traditional definition that focuses on the geographic location, face-to-face gathering, and the proximity of the community and a changing definition that allows groups of people who share interests to "gather" in well-defined online spaces (Bakardjieva, 2007; Robins, 2007).

Although the debate over whether to expand the concept of community continues, theorists do acknowledge that online communities exist. More than thirty years ago, theorists proposed "community without propinquity" (Walmsley, 2000)—a concept that would allow communities to spread out but continue to be centered on shared ideas and interests. (The term "community without propinquity" is not well phrased, as *propinquity* can mean nearness of blood [next of kin], location, or time ["propinquity," n.d.].) Online communities depend on the expanding technology and the Internet and are requiring that theorists define how the nature and perception of community are changing.

A variety of terms and definitions exist for online community. Theorists have used terms like *virtual community* and *cybercommunity* to refer to groups that meet and interact online. The term *cybercommunity* allows for community to be the best social classification and metaphor for the social interaction that involves computer-mediated communication (Fernbeck, 1999), specifically when a group meets online because of a shared purpose to interact about that purpose. (The term may be less used because of the relation of the prefix *cyber* to specific terms like *cyberpunk*, *cybercrime*, and *cyberbullying*; some scholars believe that the term *cybercommunity* is outdated.)

The greatest source of conflict regarding a definition of online communities appears to center around the virtual existence of the groups—that is, the lack of a geographic location and the characteristics that result from location—and the most frequent argument against a definition of online groups as communities (as stated earlier) is the inclusion of virtual spaces as geography, requiring geographic proximity (Bowman-Grieve, 2009) as one element that defines community. Members of online communities meet (synchronously or asynchronously) through virtual networking and maintain social connections in their online spaces; however, because those connections may result from a desire to escape reality, theorists deny that online communities meet the geography requirement. This reasoning denies the fact that some online communities are made up of members who are unable to meet geographically because they live too far apart to travel and meet or they are physically unable to travel, yet they "gather." If online communities that bear other characteristics of communities are included as communities, then globalization can be integrated into the structure of community and modern resources and creative concepts are allowed in the definition of *community*:

> detraditionalization frees us from old obligations, and lets us give community a postmodern make-over. . . . Cities have become too big, too fractured, too scary—and the Internet offers a safe space to build new communities. In sum, in the face of all this disembedding, detraditionalizing, globalizing uncertainty,

> we need to find [a] new way to belong—and the Internet is on hand to provide exactly that. (Bell, 2001, pp. 96–97)

Today, face-to-face meetings create issues that were not addressed or necessary in the past—issues such as those related to safety, populations, costs, and travel. These face-to-face interactions are not required for the success of an online community (Reich, 2010)—interactions that may potentially create bias based on physical demeanor and characteristics. Instead, online communities develop as individuals connect and share values that are independent of geography's cultural context (Zancheti, 2002); these groups are "social aggregations with common values and interests [who meet] on the Internet" (Shen, Yu, and Khalifa, 2010, p. 337). The result is a democratic process—an online community centered around the individuals who participate (Coe, 1998; Ebeling, 2003; Levine, 2002; Nah, 2010) rather than the physical elements of the location or the people.

One definition includes five attributes of an online community and eliminates the physical/geographic location as a requirement:

- "purpose (i.e., content of interaction),
- place (i.e., extent of technology mediation of interaction),
- platform (i.e., design of interaction),
- population (i.e., pattern of interaction), and
- profile model (i.e., return on interaction)" (Porter, 2004, as cited in Jin, Park, and Kim, 2010, p. 587).

This definition includes *place* that could satisfy the traditionalists who require that location be a part of the definition of community. And truly, online communities do have location; each has a uniform resource locator (URL) that identifies where the online community exists. This URL may identify a chat room, a discussion board, or some other online space—the *where* for the community members to be able to locate and identify each other. That location allows the community members to find each other and eliminates the element of distance.

Distance can be determined by whether members sit in the same room or in the same building, and communities differ per more than distance. For example, communities of learning can be in online classrooms; per the Theory of Transactional Distance (Moore, 1993), created to address distance education, spaces for education house a "university of relationships [that must be] shaped around the most elementary constructs of the field [of education]—namely, the structure of instructional programmes, the interaction between learner and teachers, and the nature and degree of the self-directedness of the learner" (p. 22). The theory acknowledges that communities of learning (classrooms) can be in virtual spaces; students do not need to meet face-to-face to build community and to learn together. This theory can be applied to online communities as well, as these virtual spaces are shaped around the motivation or purpose of those who participate, the structure of the community, and the interaction and relationships between members.

All online groups will not qualify as communities, because some structured online spaces exist, not for members to "gather" around a shared purpose and to establish relationship, but for individuals to review products, post links, and answer one-time questions. These spaces do not fulfill the three required characteristics of community proposed in this chapter. But community should not be limited by geography. As I studied online communities, I noted that they share the same three common and prominent characteristics that a traditional community shares. In online communities, members share a purpose, they "co-exist" in a structured environment, and they interact with each other and build relationships. A revised definition should address these three major characteristics that both traditional and online communities share. A definition of community that involves these three characteristics is member-centric, focusing on the individuals within the group rather than on the group and only on what or where or why it exists.

The three characteristics that separate community from other groups are similar in online communities. Online communities connect around purpose, structure, and interaction and relationships.

Purpose in Online Communities

Online communities, like traditional communities, are organized around the members' shared interest or purpose. Members may be pursuing community because of a need to belong, and "there emerges a problematic essentializing of this need, which theorizes community as a 'natural' manifestation of the 'innate' human desire for association and identification—and this motif resurfaces in discussions of online communities" (Delanty, 2009, p. 96). But more frequently, community members gather in online spaces for a shared purpose.

Consider an online community that gathers people for a shared purpose. Gaia Online's main index page states, "Welcome to Gaia's forums, where millions of members gather to discuss random stuff, make new friends, complain about life, argue about nothing, laugh at dumb pictures, discuss serious issues and/or curse like sailors. Come join in already!" (Main Index—Forum: Gaia Online, n.d.). This purpose draws people who desire to belong. However, the community has a more focused purpose: on the homepage, Gaia specifically states, "Founded in 2003, Gaia Online has grown into one of the biggest forum communities in the world. Today, Gaia is the best place on the web *to discuss anime, games, comics, sci-fi, fantasy and anything else you can imagine*" [emphasis added] (Welcome—Gaia Online, 2016). This community is successful and growing: in November 2011, the community boasted 1,987,554,803 articles posted with 25,388,484 registered users, and by December 2016, the community counted 2,336,354,591 articles with 29,653,935 registered users (Welcome—Gaia Online, 2016). The community also keeps a live count on synchronous active users, which peaked at 532,396 on March 27, 2014 (Welcome—Gaia Online, 2016). Gaia draws members with a shared purpose but allows members to break into sub-communities based on the members' specific interests and to post in various forums. Groups like Gaia Online that house members who gather online to discuss purposes are not always communities, just as groups that gather face-to-face are not always communities. Shoppers in line at a convenience store to buy lottery tickets are not a community; they may share a purpose—to buy lottery tickets—and they are in the same place, but they do not interact and build relationship.

This section would be incomplete without a reference to members who gather for shared medical or health purposes. For example, in the discussion board for BreastFeeding.com, mothers join around the shared interest of breastfeeding. The community exists to connect members—typically mothers and proponents of breastfeeding—so they can learn and share experiences. BreastFeeding.com forums include groups (subsets of the greater community) that focus on breastfeeding as well as parenting children of different ages, weight loss, cooking, and shopping (most related to breastfeeding). Similar to the well-known La Leche League (a face-to-face community with a complementary online community at www.illi.org) where women gather to learn, to act, and to support breastfeeding (Koerber, 2005), the community within BreastFeeding.org focuses on empowering women who share the purpose of breastfeeding, with a posted disclaimer that shares the purpose: "All material provided at BreastFeeding.com is provided for educational purposes only. Consult with your lactation consultant or health care provider regarding the advisability of any opinions or recommendations with respect to your individual situation" (Bump, 2011a). The shared purpose is education about breastfeeding, not to replace the expertise provided by lactation or medical experts. Other communities similarly focus on medically related interests or diagnoses such as leukemia, autism, heart disease, infertility, and cancer. (Chapter 3 will expand this discussion.)

Structure in Online Communities

Online communities exist in a structured environment—a determined virtual space where members may be required to pay a fee, register for the site, or create a profile. Some sites are created and regulated by administrators; others are maintained by corporations or by members. Most online communities abide by established expectations that govern the organization and impose expectations on the members of that community. Online communities without boundaries to identify appropriate behavior frequently will experience problems or "die" (Dumont and Candler, 2005). Therefore, online communities frequently have guidelines that include "shared social codes" (Bell, 2001, p. 100) or "netiquette" (Radin, 2006) that establishes expectations and behaviors expected of members. (Bell states that netiquette is "the less 'extreme' end of this spectrum" of "modes of social control" [p. 103] to regulate behavior within the community. Bell's narrative about multi-user domains and control of transgressions in online communities is beyond the scope of this book but is still related and interesting.)

One cannot write about structure in online communities without considering these virtual worlds and cases where the expectations of membership did not exist or were violated. One such online community was LambdaMOO, a text-based environment (a virtual mansion) where a diverse group of avatars gathered to play one Monday evening and when one member, using a voodoo programming command, raped and violated several members in the MOO (Dibbell, 1993). The MOO (a multi-user domain, object oriented) for many became a case to study the social ramifications of online communities lacking structure. The community owned the physical representation of the structure of a large mansion with multiple rooms and closets with portals into the online space, but the community had no organizational structure to address the expected behaviors of members; members anticipated that the laws, mores (customs and habits), and social expectations that exist in the physical world would be understood in a virtual world like LambdaMOO. The virtual space is described as a house or city with multiple locations, all described by words, and a diverse participating population (Coe, 1998) and members have voiced guidelines, but the technical creators of the MOO did not document, formalize, or enforce community behavior expectations:

> Allow the MOO "community" (the quotes are intended) to become what it already is: many different, overlapping and STRANGE communities/entities/groups/loose associations/whatever. Any group which [*sic*] wishes to "constitute" itself as a body with its own culture, rules, guidelines, or spiritual inclinations should be allowed to stake out a circumscribed piece of MOO "territory" for themselves [*sic*]. (10 December 1992, post #568 on *social issues; as cited by Coe, 1998, p. 398)

The online rape occurred in March 1993 (Roberts, 1999)—between this post and Dibbell's (1993) descriptive blog post of what happened that night and in the following days as the community sought to decide what penalty to impose on the rapist, Mr. Bungle. (See also Hess, 2003, for information about MOOs, online etiquette, and the LambdaMOO case.) The 1992 *social issues post (cited by Coe, 1998) stated that new groups in LambdaMOO should establish rules as part of the cultural elements that would characterize any new community. Coe (1998) commented:

> Having common rules seemed to be a mark of community. In 1994, Wheat said: "But we are not a community if we abdicate any attempt to collectively enforce some outer boundaries of behavior" (5 July 1994, post #187 on *p:disbandmediation). Lettuce, in the debate about a rule legislating a minimum punishment for MOO-rape, wrote, "There are behavioral rules for inclusion in any community. Without rules there can be no community. There don't have to be many, but they have to work" (8 May 1994, post #99 on *p:antirape). For these two MOOers, becoming a community meant not only [to] have a common space but also instituting [*sic*] common grounds of behavior." (p. 399)

Online communities create standards that reflect those of face-to-face communities, and members such as these members believe that standards in an online community are a must.

An online community also needs structure and guidelines to establish the liability limitations of the founders of the community and to ensure that members know their and the community founders' responsibilities. Community structure may incorporate disclaimers that eliminate the community founders' responsibilities for the information that members share, the way members behave, and the way that visitors use the data that members share. This structure may also include rules that direct members on the expectations for conduct in the online community—for example, *netiquette* can refer to expected behavior of members, and these expectations may overlap between the responsibilities of the community founders as well as expected cultural norms for the community.

Communities created by organizations or corporations typically alleviate issues in these online communities by establishing membership guidelines and expectations before members join the community. For example, Breast-Feeding.com houses a page for Terms & Conditions (Bump, 2011b) to which members must agree when they register to join the community, and Breast-Feeding.com's administration reserves the right to remove members who violate the conditions. The conditions include a disclaimer as well as instructions on how members are to present themselves, communicate, and behave in the community space, including that members

- must provide accurate information to register and may only use their own accounts;
- may not use the community for financial gain; and
- may not share any material that is "unlawful, harassing, libelous, defamatory, abusive, threatening, or otherwise objectionable" (Bump, 2011b).

BreastFeeding.com requires accuracy but does not ensure members' accuracy or accept liability for any consequences that members experience from using the site. These guidelines have a legal, formal tone and include standards to protect community members as well as the creators of the site.

Get Satisfaction is "a community of real people who collaborate on answers, solutions, and ideas about the products and services they love—and the ones they wish were better" (Muller, 2016). The Community Rules—"as few as possible"—are stated simply and in an informal tone with descriptions to expand the community expectations:

- Be your awesome self.
- Win friends and influence people.
- Tell it like it is.
- Have (good, clean) fun!
- Be constructive with your criticism.
- Spread the wealth.
- No hawking!
- Don't be naughty.
- Be fruitful, but don't multiply.
- No trolls!
- Those boots were made for walking.

These community rules (Muller, 2016) require authenticity, respect, frequent interaction, kindness, focus, and respect for privacy (paras. 2–12). The rules are posted by co-founder and director of community education, who adds a friendly note at the end:

> Thank you for considering these rules, which are, themselves, carefully considered. As with any community, it's up to each of us to create and participate in open conversations that can bring us together—and sometimes tear us apart. Our hope is that by sharing our passions we will grow more passionate, more wily, maybe even a little crazy, but we always pledge to be engaged and open to other voices. (Muller, 2016)

The guidelines establish standards as well as repercussions for members who violate these, giving the community administrator power to remove community members who do not comply.

The question arises: Does true community exist if the founders establish the rules? Although this question is beyond the scope of this book, the question is relevant because it does relate to the topic. In the LambdaMOO discourse, the lack of community rules allows the unthinkable to happen; however, the members rally to try to establish guidelines and expectations and formalize those. Because the communities that gather and interact within LambdaMOO are diverse, each community needs to establish its own guidelines. However, on Get Satisfaction and Gaia Online, the standards are established before the community members begin to use the space, and the structure helps the community members focus on their shared purpose rather than on creating the structure of the community. Therefore, the characteristic requires structure rather than limiting who can create the structure of the community.

Interaction in Online Communities

The members of online communities gather to interact—to send and receive messages and create relationship through discourse. Like the introduction of the telephone, which allows individuals to communicate across distances, and of the cellular phone, which allows individuals to carry the communication tool anywhere with access (Stewart, 2010), the Internet and the resulting communities eliminate issues of distance and time, limiting users only to issues related to system connections (hardware, software, and access to the Internet).

Text-based communication allows groups to interact. Researchers are asking if people who exchange messages in online spaces form real relationships and thus communities (Joinson and Dietz-Yhler, 2002, p. 275). But other researchers are finding that eliminating the geographic barriers can actually help groups create more fulfilling and intimate relationships:

> Because the forums are text-based, participants value each other on the basis of written contributions rather than physical appearance and they can carefully formulate messages for discussing emotional issues. The option to post anonymous messages facilitates discussion of sensitive topics. Last, the wide reach of forums provides access to an expanded network of peers who communicate across barriers of time and location. (Hwang, Ottenbacher, Lucke, et al., 2011, p. 199)

Text-based communication allows members to think ahead and eliminates physical complications and biases that might influence how a group in a geographically founded community accepts a member. Instead, individuals communicate via text in a computer-mediated setting (Want, Chen, and Tsai, 2012) without the complications of demographics, appearances, and other body-based biases. These online groups "transform previously impassable barriers to communication into permeable lines of differentiation because the channels of the Internet are not constrained by traditional borders" (Kotowski and dos Santos, 2010, p. 152). These researchers theorize that if the Internet is acknowledged as a location and a group has other characteristics of a community, then an online community is just that—a community.

One important question about membership and belonging in an online community is what one must do to be part of a community. Community members on a music-focused discussion board discussed this, and Active (2010) summed up several members' comments:

> isn't that the fun of communities? and real, progressive communities? no one is trying to take advantage of anyone, there are no real "leaders" and no real "followers". just people who exist and share together. and as pauk said, when we do venture beyond our cubicles in cities, homes in suburbs, or diamond incrusted mansions with butlers, er manservants, tigers, hot tubs, and more cars then most dictators and rockstars ever could imagine (aka home in the mountains), we meet on the same plain: inspired people creating and sharing art. (para. 1)

Antiphon (2010, October 29) replied "I lurked for many months and the first time I posted I was nervous, thinking I didn't really have anything substantial to contribute. I still don't think I do, but I have been treated warmly and fairly here, and that is enough to make me feel like I belong" (para. 3). According to members, community requires that you interact and that you feel like you belong because you are interacting. As members showed their commitment to the community by interacting, "they accrue social trust and a positive reputation" that encourages other members to participate and thus leads the cybercommunity to succeed (Huffaker, 2010, p. 596) and helps members to build their relationships (Wenger, 2006).

Critics of online communities as *communities* emphasize that the *lack* of physical closeness is not only beneficial but also necessary for groups that function as communities (Bakardijev, 2007; Robins, 2007). However, as technology becomes a means for interaction, geography becomes less of an issue for individuals who desire to be part of a community. "Belonging has been radically reshaped, leading many to question the very possibility of belonging as it disappears into the flow of communication. The result is that place, locality and symbolic ties are being drained of any content. In their place are more fluid and temporary forms of social relations sustained only by processes of communication outside of which they have no reality" (Delanty, 2010, p. 135). As a result, "community is defined by feelings of trust, respect, or relationship" (West, 2010, p. 70), rather than geography, proximity, and physical access. Community members can create relationships without a face-to-face element. As a result, they may not interact outside the community space; they substitute a virtual space for geography but interact as they would in a traditional community.

In the same way, in online communities, members need to interact to know each other, as they cannot identify each other per physical characteristics like they can in face-to-face communities. However, there are those individuals, called *lurkers*, who visit the community and view interactions but do not participate. Per lurkers, researchers disagree on their role: for example, Liu (1999) states that lurkers are not a part of an online community because, "for a group of individuals to qualify as a community, these individuals have to communicate and interact" (para. 29). He justifies his decision to omit lurkers as a part of the community (and thus a part of his research of a community), justifying the omission by stating that lurkers could influence his findings and create misleading results; however, because he measured community interaction, the lurkers are not a part of that action. Similarly, Steinmetz (2012), an ethnographer, denies lurkers as players in online communities, stating that lurkers, who are nonparticipants, are insignificant in the actions within a community because lurkers are not visibly present and thus do not directly influence the community; "[lurkers] are only relevant if the community makes them relevant" (p. 32).

In contrast, other researchers acknowledge a rule for lurkers in a community. For example, Yeh, Lin, and Lu (2011) label *lurker* as a role that some individuals play within the community and thus include lurkers when the researchers poll community members, noting that lurkers participate to "create enjoyable experiences through observation" (p. 763). Similarly, Riding, Gefen, and Arinze (2006) include lurkers, stating that they are desirable because they create balance and ensure against information overload (p. 331) as well as serve as the advertisers' audiences, the traffic in an online community, and a quantifiable part of the server volume (p. 330). Members of a community recognize that lurkers exist and consider them as a positive part of the community (Merry and Simon, 2012). In fact, 26 percent of U.S. adults who use the Internet report that, in the last year, they have watched online someone else's health or medical experiences, and 16 percent state that they went online to find someone who shares the same health concerns (Fox and Duggan, 2013). However, they didn't interact. Lurkers must be addressed in a discussion of the elements of an online community because they too must abide by and submit themselves to the structure of the community. However, lurkers do not add to the interaction and relationships built within a community.

Because online communities do not identify membership—attendance is difficult to verify because non-participatory members are not easily tracked—interaction is particularly relevant for online communities. Members create singular or multiplexed "ties" (Garton, Haythornthwaite, and Wellman, 1997). But technology creates flexibility in those ties, allowing community members to decide when, where, and how they interact and to invest in the community and relationships and thus to define how they bond with regard to a shared purpose:

> Strong ties that are on-line have many characteristics that are similar to strong off-line ties. They encourage *frequent*, *companionable* contact and are *voluntary* except in work situations. One or two keystrokes are all that is necessary to begin replying, facilitating *reciprocal*, *mutual support* of tie partners' needs.

> Moreover, the placelessness of email contacts aids *long-term* contact, without the loss of the tie that so often accompanies geographical mobility. (Wellman and Gulia, 1999, p. 10)

In the same way, relationships via other media (such as instant messages, chat rooms, and discussion boards) allow for that long-term contact and communication related to a shared purpose or interest and thus allow for the maintenance and strengthening of those distanced ties.

When members of online communities do not interact, the community dies (Dumont and Candler, 2005; Iriberri and Leroy, 2009). To interact successfully, members must participate in the culture of the community and be able to share rhetoric—the language of that culture. The members must speak the same language, which may be related to geographic culture and nationality but may also relate to the culture of the specific online community. Posts can contain terms that are unique to the community as well as to online communities because of the virtual space where the community exists. (For example, consider the reference to "No trolls!" from earlier in chapter 1; the term *troll* has adapted from its use in face-to-face community to that in online community.) Members must *speak* within the online space—text-based communication, as mentioned earlier—whether on discussion boards, blogs, forums, chat rooms, listservs, or other virtual settlements (Jones, 1997). Additionally, the members' language must be meaningful so members can converse about the topic they are discussing (Gallagher, 2009)—so members can communicate. This "communication is the medium in which belonging is today being expressed in its most important ways. This leads to the argument that virtual communities are only one form of community and that they exist alongside other kinds of community" (Bell, 2001, p. 135). In fact, because members of online communities cannot implement nonverbal communication but instead depend on aural or visual presentations of language (through recorded or text-based communication), online communities become "one of the best examples we have of communication communities, because one aim of the virtual community is the sharing of information" (Bell, 2001, p. 137). Member interaction is communication with (mostly) text, so members must use emerging media—technology—to effectively and efficiently communicate. They must also consider the language they use because communication in some media (such as discussion boards and forums) is asynchronous and thus allows time between exchanges of discourse.

Communication can be empty, but interaction builds relationships; consistent, personal, effective rhetoric is the key to establishing and maintaining viable relationships (whether in real life or in virtual spaces), and collective relationships in a shared online settlement create community. Online relationships allow for the review of the rhetoric before it is published for the other person to see. For that reason, online discourse allows individuals to think before they speak in the community—a benefit that can help them to submit more effective and efficient messages. In addition, online relationships can allow for greater intimacy because "on-line messages can be sent at any time and to anyone and can be responded to when time is available. This level of access does not transfer to face-to-face situations where different social, personal, and community rules exist" (Costigan, 1999, p. xxii). Online relationships therefore are convenient and thus sometimes easier for those involved. Through this interaction, members create an emotional attachment as well as a sense of belonging where "members [feel] that this [is] a space in which they [are] free to discuss feelings openly and in the process develop bonds with other members" (O'Connor and Mackeogh, 2007, p. 103), exchanging information (Matzat, 2010; Xia, Huant, Duan, and Whinston, 2009) and conversing regularly (Wenger, 2006).

DISCOURSE IN THE ONLINE COMMUNITY

When individuals communicate with each other, they discourse. *Discourse* is a nominalization derived from Latin and French that describes the act of involved parties as they converse, reason, think, and understand (discourse, n.d.). But discourse is even more complicated:

> The notion of discourse encompasses, at the macro level, kinds of knowledge that regulate our thinking, such as discourses of pain or sexuality. At the most micro level, it includes the largely unconscious ways in which we process text and talk. This breadth allows for many different approaches to discourse analysis . . . including discursive psychology and conversation analysis. (Roberts and Sarangi, 2005, p. 632)

Discourse is the complex action of two or more individuals communicating with the undercurrent of who they are and what and how they think. The act of discourse requires two or more parties who are reasoning and interacting to share information and to understand each other. Their messages are relayed with the intent to transfer information from one party to another and to persuade each other to respond. To learn about discourse and the behaviors related to human interaction and communication, researchers identify the purpose of that discourse, focus the studies, and gather and analyze data. Through their studies, researchers are able to

- answer questions related to communication and human interaction,
- solve communication problems by testing options, and
- test and expand what already exists in the corpus of knowledge about the topic.

As they assess their findings, researchers can create new theories that relate to their research. They can better understand humans, anticipate future behaviors, and identify trends. Specifically, research of these online communities can investigate

- what members are discussing,
- what resources and information they share,
- how members support each other,
- how they perceive the online community, and
- how members construct their narratives and establish membership in these online communities.

Research of these online texts should "illuminate texts while . . . using texts to illuminate, deepen, and refine understanding of the sensitizing concepts" (Gill and Babrow, 2010, p. 138). In other words, in considering discourse in online communities, research should focus on community texts and allow the voices of the community members to speak and to create theoretical frameworks, and, in considering questions related to human behavior and communication, researchers must carefully design studies to investigate relevant data using appropriate and effective methods. But researchers must also keep the humanity of community members in mind in designing studies and analyzing data. The ethical complications and choices related to discourse (some of which are discussed in chapter 4) must be considered so the humans involved in the discourse and their rights are respected.

The rhetoric on a discussion board includes language that applies to the community's focus and location—words, phrases, interaction, and ideas that relate to the community's space and topic. On the discussion board of Breastcancer.org, the members use terms related to medicine and breast cancer but their discourse also includes online terms. For example, one member addresses the members participating in the "Progesterone Cream" thread when she asks a question and then states,

> I am not being a troll, I am trying to wrap my hands around a lot of information in a short time frame (Gwenn).

Troll is a slang term for someone who enters an online space or community (such as an online game, a chat room, or discussion board) with the intent to disrupt the interaction in that space (O'Connor and Mackeogh, 2007; Turner, 2009). Gwenn expresses that she is not a troll because she wants to ask a medically focused question, but as a newcomer to the thread, she does not want the other members to think that her intent is to disrupt the discourse in their conversation.

(I must note that the administrators of Breastcancer.org follow the interaction within the discussion board and remove trolls' posts. In fact, in one thread that I analyzed, the administrators removed a post, evidenced by a notation of a removed post and by the comments around the missing post by the community members who saw the post before it was removed. I am unaware of why the administration removed the post, but shortly after the note of removal, one of the members posted a thank you to the administrators.)

Other members integrate technology-specific language into their discourse. For example, members use "LOL," an abbreviation created for texting that means "laugh out loud." Other members use similar terms that relate to online spaces: "cyberfriends" (Melissa), "TMI" (too much information; Jeanne), and several emoticons and "(((HUGS)))" (with the parentheses imitating the arms of a person giving a hug). Some elements of the discourse within this online community are specific to online and digital communication.

The members also understand the mechanics of the online space and can manipulate the mechanics to serve the members of the thread. For example, one member (Valinda) posts a greeting to the women who are participating in the thread and then explains that she is posting to keep the thread at the top of the list of active threads on the Breastcancer.org homepage. (The homepage contains an abbreviated list of threads on which members have most recently posted, so Valinda is seeking to pull the thread to the top of that active list to keep the thread visible to the overall community and thus encourage other members to join the discourse.) Her explanation illustrates how she thinks in regard to recruiting new participation in threads of discourse and how she understands the mechanics of how the discussion board technically works. By explaining, she is also educating other members so they too can act to bring the thread to the top of the list of active threads.

The members recognize that they are interacting in an online community. Knowing the community's "location," they act per the mechanics of the technology and also allow their language to reflect the online space. Their discourse then is relevant to the fact that they are interacting online.

Discourse within a community benefits those who are participating on a variety of levels. The community benefits as a whole when the individuals participate (Delanty, 2010; Rheingold, 1993) because the individuals who share their stories help the group to grow in perspective, potential skill and action, knowledge, and diversity that strengthens the group as a whole. Participants also benefit positively as individuals. In this environment, the participants fellowship (Arduser, 2011, p. 6) and experience connection, something they are seeking in a community. And other participants benefit when members share positive experiences and narratives; these narratives share joy and hope.

Participants who share negative stories also benefit from the story-telling process. When these individuals share negative experiences, particularly traumatic experiences, that expression benefits them physically and psychologically. Individuals experience fewer health problems when they communicate—via written and oral narratives—about traumatic experiences because they eliminate stress related to not confronting trauma (e.g., Pennebaker, 1993; Pennebaker, Kiecolt-Glaser, and Glaser, 1988). *Traumatic* relates to *trauma*: "serious injury to the body, as from physical violence or an accident; severe emotional or mental distress caused by an experience; an experience that causes severe anxiety or emotional stress, such as rape or combat (and memories that persist after a trauma occurs). An event or situation that causes great disruption or suffering" ("traumatic," n.d.). Pennebaker finds that individuals who write about traumatic experiences—those that create severe emotional duress—report more positive attitudes, and his research shows that those individuals who disclose more about their experiences gain greater health benefits (Pennebaker, Kiecolt-Glaser, and Glaser, 1988). Additionally, in *Forming a Story: The Health Benefits of Narrative*, Pennebaker and Seagal (1999) report "Extensive research has revealed that when people put their emotional upheavals into words, their physical and mental health improves markedly" (p. 1244). Other research finds that these trauma narratives help those involved to recover and is "a principle that is common to most trauma intervention models" (Kaminer, 2006, p. 481). Individuals benefit from sharing their experiences.

Additional research suggests that people who participate in online communities benefit because they share their feelings and sources of stress (Beaudoin and Tao, 2007; Rodgers and Chen, 2005). They also experience connection with others who share their experiences. Participation in the communication process is beneficial.

For a community that focuses on a medical diagnosis, the members benefit from sharing their illness narratives. An illness narrative is the story of a patient's experience through the disease process. Although some illness narratives are maintained by healthcare professionals and family members on behalf of patients during critical care (Egerod, Christensen, Schwartz-Nielsen, and Agard, 2011) and thus are biographical in tone, they are more frequently autobiographical (first-person) accounts of patients' experiences (Garden, 2010; Hinson, 2016) shared through a variety of media including journals, Web logs, and discussion-board posts. These illness narratives are valuable to the rhetorics of health and medicine; these narratives provide researchers and scholars with authentic experiential accounts of illness, a valuable venue for patient voices and agency to be considered.

MEMBERS IN ONLINE COMMUNITIES

Members in online communities are individuals who have Internet access and who simultaneously connect (Milson, 2002) because they share a purpose. Some of those connections are nontraditional, socially deviant, unique, or sensitive issues, and members are dispersed geographically and cannot access each other: "There may be only a handful of practitioners of an unusual hobby, or sufferers of a rare illness, in any given community, denying the group both the critical mass to interact and the ability, like needles in a haystack, to identify each other" (Dumont and Candler, 2005). Online communities allow these individuals to gather and interact, creating relationships and sharing when face-to-face society might create discomfort or rejection. Examples include individuals who are pro–eating disorders (McCabe, 2009); Africa-descended populations who are historically dispersed (Ebeling, 2003); individuals living with limiting physical disabilities (Obst and Stafurik, 2010); intersexed individuals (Still, 2008); and online terrorist supporters (Bowman-Grieve, 2009). Members of these organizations cannot or will not meet in face-to-face environments, and online communities provide them with a safe, comfortable environment where they can meet and interact.

The online community may also develop because few individuals share the interest and these few can find each other online: "Where I lived then in Memphis and now in St. Louis, there are few others in the immediate neighborhood who share my deep interest in. . . . The list [a discussion list] allowed me to connect immediately with a community of kindred souls and then to keep that community when I changed locations. . . . I believe the . . . on-line community is a good example" (Kruse, 1998, p. 5). This member of an online community acknowledges that the group allows her to share her interest and interact with others in a structured (discussion-list) environment. Thus, these groups are structured online organisms that develop around the members and their interests.

In some communities, including Breastcancer.org, two types of people visit the publically published content. The first type, *members*, are individuals who have registered so they can have the privilege to participate, and the second are *visitors*, who are not registered. Members are men and women who have created accounts and profiles in the Website database: each member registers an email address, creates a username and a signature, shares demographic information, and agrees to abide by the community guidelines as they participate. After registering, members can post and participate in the chat rooms or on the discussion board.

Visitors do not register but, in communities like Breastcancer.org that are not password protected and thus are public communities, they can access the community content, which is available to anyone who has access to the space through the World Wide Web. Visitors cannot post and do not receive outside communication from Breastcancer.org. (Communication scholars ask if visitors should be considered a part of an online community, a question that should be considered in future research.)

Breastcancer.org seeks to provide members with a space that allows patients to interact, sometimes when they might not feel like a face-to-face meeting. Because they are not able to dress to attend, they feel self-conscious about their silhouette of healing amputated breasts and bald heads, or they are unable to move because chemotherapy-caused nausea and damaged tissue creates discomfort and incredible pain. Thus, an online community like Breastcancer.org provides "a secure and supportive place to interact with others who will provide nonjudgmental support" (McCabe, 2009, p. 3) to "forge new, virtual communities that previously may not have been possible without the aid of the Internet" (Ebeling, 2003, p. 101) and thus to improve the members' personal networks (Hwang, Ottenbacher, Lucke, et al., 2011) and well-being (Obst and Stafurik, 2010). Breastcancer.org seeks to inform members on the structure of the community and thus acknowledges in the community guidelines (Breastcancer.org.—Community Guidelines, 2016) that the site content is publicly available, and the Breastcancer.org homepage for the community (Breastcancer.org Community, 2016) documents the number of posts as well as the number of views that each thread receives.

PATIENT-CENTERED ONLINE COMMUNITIES

As communication changes, health communication is shifting:

- to allow interaction between healthcare professionals and patients,
- to give patients more immediate access to general health information and empower them to participate in their medical care,
- to adapt to emerging media and the digital spaces that patients and providers are using, and
- to allow for more authentic and transparent discourse related to health and wellness.

As health information is more readily accessible, health communication allows all stakeholders to participate: for example, physicians can write descriptions of disease and treatments for medically focused Websites; nonprofits can inform their audiences about research and raise funds online; nutritionalists and dieticians can share information and healthy diets; trainers can instruct their audiences about exercise regimens; and patients can interact and share experiences with others via online communities.

Online communities focus on a variety of medical disorders and health-related topics and are thriving because non–medically trained members have questions to ask, support to seek, and experiences to share with others who have the same concerns or diagnoses. Online communities have developed around groups interested in a variety of disorders and medical needs. Some frequent purposes include autism, breastfeeding, cancer, depression, diabetes, and HPV:

- Autism/PDD Information and Support to Help Your Child (http://www.autism-pdd.net) exists to provide support for those with and family members with autism spectrum disorders.
- The BreastFeeding.Com Community (http://www.breastfeeding.com/forums) exists for breastfeeding mothers to share experiences, to ask questions, and to communicate about every-day life with other mothers who value breastfeeding.
- Cancer Survivors Network (http://csn.cancer.org/forum) provides a list of cancer-specific discussion boards on which individuals confronting specific cancers can communicate about their diseases.
- Depression Message Board & Forum Discussions: HealthBoards (http://www.healthboards.com/boards/depression) allows those who suffer from or live with someone who suffers from depression to share their stories and to gain advice and support from others in similar situations.
- Diabetic Connect (http://www.diabetescommunity.com) provides a place for diabetics to interact and to gather information.
- HPV Support—HPV/Genital Warts Support Community (http://www.hpvsupport.com/phpBB3) provides people living with the Human Papilloma Virus (HPV) with an online community where they can discuss their feelings, experiences, treatments, and personal stories.

Disease and illness are not occurrences that patients visit once; they may live with a chronic disease and thus need long-term (even life-long) relationships with others who are empathetic to strive, thrive, and survive their diseases.

The list of online communities that focus on health and medical diagnoses is almost endless; in fact, a search on Google of "health online community" in June 2017 resulted in 593 million pages in 0.45 seconds. In these online communities, individuals gather because of a shared medical diagnoses or health concern in a structured environment to interact about their experiences and concerns as they support each other and create relationships. Many of these sites include "community" in their URLs and in their page names but they are communities per the definition I propose: they are groups of members with a shared purpose who exist in an established virtual space with various regulations and standards who interact and thus create a "slice of life" online (Jones, 1999b, p. 12).

Researchers are investigating these medically focused online communities as more Americans use the Internet to find medical information (Blank and Adams-Blodnieks, 2007; Orgad, 2005; Segal, 2005; Still, 2008). Members of these online communities receive support, hope, and disease-specific information in these communities, and they also access these online communities to learn about their options and treatments (Shah and Robinson, 2011)—such as time-saving methods and money-saving tips as well as how to use equipment, how to communicate with their healthcare providers, and how to pay for treatment—as well as how to advocate (Still, 2009, p. 47).

Online communities focused on breast cancer are frequently springing up on the Internet because breast cancer is the most frequently diagnosed disease for women (Lichtenfeld, 2010) and affects 1 in 8 women annually in the United States. (National Cancer Institute, n.d.b.) as well as their family members and friends. The rate of diagnosis in the United States is reported to be decreasing (Bandi, Brinton, Buchert, et al., 2009) or at least plateauing (Ravdin, Cronin, Howlader, et al., 2003), but breast cancer is still a deadly threat for women. As women are diagnosed, many are visiting online sites and online communities to cope, to learn, to survive, and to thrive. They are using online sources to learn about their diagnoses and participating in online communities to interact and discourse with other women about the disease. A search on Google for "breast cancer community" in June 2017 returned 74 million results in 0.41 seconds. These findings included

- Breastcancer.org (http://www.Breastcancer.org);
- National Breast Cancer Foundation, Inc. (http://www.nationalbreastcancer.org);
- Advanced Breast Cancer Community (http://www.advancedbreastcancercommunity.org);
- Revolution Health—Breast Cancer Community (http://www.revolutionhealth.com/community-overview/cancer/breast-cancer);
- WebMD Breast Cancer Community (http://exchanges.webmd.com/breast-cancer-exchange);
- Friends in Need Breast Cancer Support Forum (http://www.friendsinneed.com); and
- Breast Cancer Support (http://bcsupport.org).

These communities focus on individuals who have been diagnosed with breast cancer and are all public communities (that is, content is not protected by passwords). Although the members of these online communities share concerns about breast cancer, they interact about more than only their disease; as they invest more and interact more in the community, they share life. "Many women view their own experiences as important sources of information that should be shared with each other. The Internet offers breast cancer survivors a plethora of ways to 'seek connections.' . . . These include listservs, e-mail and chat rooms, but also the network of personal web pages. . . .

The intersections of all of these have created what many see as a virtual community" (Pitts, 2004, p. 46). Discussion boards are also emerging media that house virtual communities—for "the sharing of information, advice and support, but also for the airing of women's embodied experiences of sickness, healing, recovery, mourning and survival" (Pitts, 2004, p. 49), where these women generate "new forms of knowledge, awareness and agency in relation to the illness" (Pitts, 2004, p. 34). These online spaces truly do provide a structured place where members can gather to interact about a shared purpose.

Online communities focusing on breast cancer can empower patients, provide them with support and information as well as companionship, and allow them to be whole rather than only patients in every interaction related to their diseases. Members interacting in these online communities are sharing their narratives (Orgad, 2005), through which they express personal agency and are empowered to control the disease process. They can also advocate together to make a difference. (For example, BCANS, an online community centered in the United Kingdom, works to improve the lives of some of their most needy members [Radin, 2006].) These online communities also offer 24/7 interactivity without the geographic boundaries that limit who can meet and interact with what patients and they thus shatter "the information monopoly" (Radin, 2006, p. 600) that patients sometimes feel with their healthcare providers. Members use online communities to

- obtain information from others (Anderson and Klemm, 2008; Dickerson, Boemhmke, Ogle, and Brown, 2006);
- discuss new treatments (Bradley, 2008; Dickerson, Boemhmke, Ogle, and Brown, 2006);
- communicate about their side effects and symptoms (Im, Chee, Lim, et al., 2007); and
- relate to others with breast cancer (Beaudoin and Tao, 2007; Bradley, 2008; Im, Chee, Lim, et al., 2007).

Members of online communities participate in these virtual spaces in a variety of ways.

COMMUNITY VIA BREASTCANCER.ORG

Breastcancer.org is the largest American-based online community that focuses on breast cancer. Created by an oncologist in 1999, the Website and online community were created "to address the need for accessible, understandable, and compassionate information about breast cancer treatment issues" (About Breastcancer.org, 2016, para. 1). Since its inception, Breastcancer.org has grown into a nonprofit organization with a board of directors and a staff (Breastcancer.org Team, 2016) and has built more than eight thousand pages of information (About Breastcancer.org, 2016). As part of the organization, Breastcancer.org contains a community with a discussion board; the community can be accessed by anyone via the homepage through the Internet to view posts, but members must register to participate on the pages. The page labeled "Community" takes a visitor to the discussion board. Membership of the community is growing: from 116,793 members in July 2012, to 183,168 members in February 2017, a 64 percent increase in almost five years.

The description of the community at Breastcancer.org invites visitors to

- participate with a purpose (to read what others have posted),
- join a structured place (this online support group), and
- interact (submit your questions).

Members in this online community gather because of a shared purpose in a structured environment to interact and create relationships.

Purpose in Breastcancer.org

Breastcancer.org exists as an online community for men and women who have been diagnosed with breast cancer—to interact, share information, support others and gain support, and provide information. "Not only is the concept of a community a 'construct' (model), it is a 'sociological construct.' [Community] is a set of interactions, human behaviours that have meaning and expectations between its members. Not just action, but actions based on sharing expectations, values, beliefs and meanings between individuals" (Bartle, 2007, para. 7). This online community brings together patients with the purpose of surviving and thriving through breast cancer. None of them want to be in a community focused on breast cancer; in fact, a common sentiment from members is "I'm sorry that you've joined us" or "I'm sorry you have to go through this." (Virginia, Mary, Hayley, Stacy, Shari, Anne, and Janie posted similar messages in the "Just Diagnosed" thread on Breastcancer.org.) The members of this online community also share secondary objectives, such as influencing care-related policy, insurance, politics, and rights in the physician–patient relationship. (In a similar online community, the women on the board petitioned that a member be reinstated to her job after she was fired because of her illness [Radin, 2006].) For example, on Breastcancer.org, Becky encourages the new members to ask physicians for second opinions, Whitney and Adrian discuss insurance issues (as do Elisabeth and Vickie), and Ashlyn and Joy advocate for less difficult treatment regimens and additional research.

Though the members are geographically separated, they relate through the purpose and the relationships within the online community. They feel a bond because they share a purpose in this community:

> I am sorry to vent here ladies, but the community site I run is for horror fans and I just cant keep talking tot hem because most of them just don't understand. So thank you for letting me vent this huge letter (Lora).

Sharing this purpose gives members credibility with each other. For example, one member posts,

> You are, indeed, in the right place! I am so sorry that you are going through this, but very glad you have found us. There are some pretty amazing women here ready to lend an ear and offer your words of encouragement and support. This is also one of the best places I have found to get information about breast cancer, its treatments, and living with the disease (Virginia).

Another member, who works in the medical field (per her introduction in her post), reiterates this community as focused on breast cancer and being a credible source:

> Come here often for support and correct information. This board [Breastcancer.org] kept me sane when I was having my chomo & rads (Ashlynn).

Other members post similar messages, indicating that, if you share the purpose as a patient with breast cancer, you have credibility within the online community. Thus, this shared purpose means more than that the members have breast cancer; it also includes the members' experiences and desires.

Structure in Breastcancer.org

Breastcancer.org is a structured environment with membership standards and requirements with community governance. The standards and requirements are posted on a page titled "Community Rules"; this page addresses behavior, expectations, and security (Breastcancer.org—Community Guidelines, 2016). In 2012, Breastcancer.org had a page called "Community Rules" and listed thirteen rules, but since then, the administration has changed the tone of the page and renamed the page to "Community Guidelines," which begins with a statement of purpose and an introduction:

> The Breastcancer.org Online Community is a service provided by Breastcancer.org to give people affected by breast cancer a place to come for support, encouragement, and commiseration. We're a welcoming community, free of judgement, and open to all who've been touched by this disease. Connect, share, learn, or just read; there is no right or wrong way to be a part of this

> place (although we strongly encourage participation—you get out what you put in). This is a Community mostly run by its members, so please keep that in mind as you find your way around; Breastcancer.org doesn't endorse or take responsibility for the content you'll find on the Discussion Boards. Our small team of moderators (mods) does keep an eye on things and are available for help or a listening ear, but our members do most of the heavy lifting to keep things welcoming and civil. As we do rely on our members to take care of the Community, we ask a few simple things in return for your membership here. If you see anything here you need clarity on, please let the mods know via private message or by emailing community@breastcancer.org.

The introduction is followed by eighteen numbered guidelines.

The administration of Breastcancer.org includes guidelines that reserves the organizations' right to governance: "Breastcancer.org reserves the right to terminate or limit your access to the Discussion Boards without notice" (Community Guidelines, 2016, Rule 17). To participate in the Breastcancer.org Community, an individual must register, create a profile, and agree to the "Community Guidelines."

Breastcancer.org establishes guidelines to protect its members as well as the administrators of the organization, and the moderators of Breastcancer.org enforce these guidelines. For example, in the "Just Diagnosed" thread, Gigi posted a message but, within 48 hours, the moderators replaced the post with "This post was deleted by Moderators." Three posts later, Beth posted, "Thank you to the moderators for deleting Gigi's post and link." With similar posts, the members of this online community acknowledge the guidelines and the moderators and appreciate the safety of this online community.

The members also formally acknowledge the cultural norms—the netiquette—for this community. For example, the "Just Diagnosed" thread was created by the moderators of Breastcancer.org to inform new members of where to find initial information about the community, but several new members began to post there. Some of the netiquette comes from experienced members: Adrian (who had already posted 8,248 posts and been in the community for 5 years) posted,

> You all will be doing better to go to the top of the page and use the 'post' to start your own thread so the other gals will know you are here. This thread was started by the monitors [moderators] just to give a little info. to help you get started. come on down to the 'meat' [the more specific threads] and you'll get lots of responses.

Ava (who had only six posts in her one month of membership) replied, "TY [Thank you]. . . . I didn't know how it worked. I appreciate it." They choose to submit to the guidelines that the administration has established, per their language. In this way, they build community in a structured environment.

Interaction in Breastcancer.org

Breastcancer.org's second note in the "Community Guidelines" (2016) says, "Say hello! Introduce yourself. Share as much or as little of your story as you're comfortable with, but please let us know you're here. That first step can be the hardest for some people, so better to jump right in. We're all here for you." This community exists to encourage interaction, and the members respond. Women ask questions and offer answers but also ask about other members' significant others, children, anniversaries, birthdays, and elements of personal lives. They laugh, share stories, and interact past their shared purpose in the online community, fulfilling five general reasons (see also Blank and Adams-Blodnieks, 2007; Orgad, 2005; Radin, 2006): to create friendships with each other, to exchange information about their medical experiences, to give and receive spiritual and emotional support, to "play" (tell jokes and play games as well as laugh at challenges and experiences), and to ask for medical and health resources.

This interaction is typical for an online community:

> For me the whole idea of "community" . . . is hard to pin down. Are people who play Farmville a community? Is a weekly book group a community? Are people who follow a particular Twitter feed a community? Are the users of a local skate park a community? In other words, when does a group of people become more than just a group of people all doing a similar thing? I'm not really sure, but mutual support and a willingness to see oneself as connected to a larger whole seems to be a start. (Antiphon, 2010, para. 2)

On Breastcancer.org, lurkers can visit the posts and gather information, but individuals must join the community to interact and to belong.

FUTURE OF ONLINE COMMUNITIES AND DISCOURSE

As technology expands and as medicine becomes more patient-centric, the number of online communities that focus on medical diagnoses will expand. Patients will continue to connect and interact through these communities. Each community will have its own culture, including its own rhetoric.

Chapter Two

The Rhetoric of Breast Cancer

Communication is the essence of being human. Humans interact to express themselves, to share information, to develop and manage data, to persuade and motivate others to act, to tell stories, to heal from traumatic experiences, and to imagine and create. Communication is integral to relationships. However, it is not specific to a particular language, style, gender, age, ethnicity, or format and instead is unique depending on a human's situation, culture, preferences, and expectations as well as the history of the circumstances and other considerations to address the audience, allow and encourage two-sided interaction, and accomplish the purpose of that interaction. Effective communication is rhetorical.

Rhetoric is constantly evolving: languages change, sentences and paragraphs shift, tools emerge, audiences and society adapt, community and values shift, and the methods that humans use to interact advance to move with those changes. Languages change as people create new words and meanings for established terms and as dictionaries acknowledge those new words. Sentence structure changes. Writing shifts as reading formats and tools evolve with technology, and signs and symbols change as communication methods and tools adapt. New tools emerge, and humans shift their communication methods: e.g., from writing with a wedge in clay to pencils on paper, to word processing that can check grammar and spelling, and to mobile devices that suggest the next words in a sentence. Audiences and society adapt as language evolves. Community and values adapt to trends in standards determined by the changing audience. And methods change; they must because people in an interacting society are consistently adapting their communication.

Even through changes, however, humans think rhetorically. "To think rhetorically is to reflect constructively on the habits of representation that position people for making judgment. Rhetoric is concerned with the invention of language that enables action, but also with the capacities of language to address and persuade" (Lyne, 2001, p. 13). Rhetoric includes *what* speakers are saying, *when* they speak and share their messages, and *how* they construct their language to inform and influence their audiences.

The digital age is affecting rhetoric. Rhetorical principles that once were considered communication elements—including tone, body language, volume, intonation, and other communication qualities that relate to verbal communication—are not relevant in text-based digital conversations. Conversely, using technology to communicate is creating new standards and requiring communication experts to interpret foundational theories through a new lens and to adapt methods to fit the rhetorical situations established in digital framework. These theories and the technology do affect how humans interact in the digital age. People seek immediate interaction through handheld tools, such as smartphones and tablets, and through applications that allow them to connect outside their previous geographic possibilities. These connections result in expanded communities and discourse with creative, unlimited conversations that reflect the relationships and the priorities of the people within the communities. These connections also reflect trends in communication, and researching helps us to observe, identify, and understand these trends and how to influence and encourage more effective communication.

In his work *Rhetoric* (written in 350 BCE), Aristotle specifies that rhetors speak in three defined situations: forensic (legal) speaking to present evidence and arguments in the courtroom, epideictic (ceremonial) speaking to memorialize or honor another person, and deliberative (political) speaking to influence decision and policy makers (Aristotle, 1924/350 BCE, Bk. I, Pt. 3, paras. 1–4). He also notes that a rhetor who is effectively speaking persuades through proofs—through the speaker's logical argument or process (*logos*) in the message, the speaker's credibility and character (*ethos*), and the emotional appeal (*pathos*) of the speaker to the audience (Aristotle, 1924/350 BCE, Bk II, Pt. 1, paras. 1–4). In addition, rhetoric involves the style and organization—i.e., effective and masterful use of language (Aristotle, 1924/350 BCE, Bk III, Pt. 1, para. 1). Therefore, rhetoric encompasses purposeful communication that focuses on the audience but addresses the topic in a manner that is authentic to the audience and to the speaker's purpose.

A rhetorical analysis of select threads from Breastcancer.org uncovers the rhetoric of breast cancer as the community members in this online community use language: to inform each other about their experiences with breast cancer, to criticize caregivers and sometimes the U.S. healthcare system, to ask each other questions and persuade other members to respond, to share resources about breast cancer that they have found in their personal research, and to accomplish other purposes. The community members discourse with each other; their intended audiences are limited to individuals who have been diagnosed with breast cancer (and sometimes with friends and family members who participate in the online community to gather information so they can take care of their loved ones). The discourse has little structured organization; the structure of the discourse depends on the initial post of each thread. The women are responding to previous posts, and the posts are published by the discussion-board program in reverse chronology, with the most recently published post first. This order allows visitors to the post to see the title and initial post of a thread and the most recent response to the conversation.

The language within these posts are informal, sometimes with incorrect mechanics (spelling, punctuation, grammar, and capitalization) and unintentional and inconsistent style. The women's intent is interaction and discourse rather than perfectly worded posts with intentional diction. The incorrect mechanics and sometimes redundant and ambiguous style reflects an immediacy of response: that is, the members may not proofread their posts and thus publish their responses with typographical or mechanical errors. Additionally, they include sentence fragments and run-ons, mixed punctuation including exclamation points, and other indicators of emotion. However, the diction does include a mixture of technical language and slang. The slang is characteristic of the informal discourse, but the technical language reflects the incredible amount of medical information that the women posting have gathered from their healthcare professionals, their friends and family, other patients who have gone through the disease process before them, their research related to their diagnoses, and other members of the community. They do repeat and affirm content, repeating information with which they agree. The rhetoric of breast cancer includes technical language but also includes slang and an informal tone that allows for incorrect sentence structure and mechanics.

These women write this way because they want to expand the safety of this Internet space (Bell, 2001), where they can openly share their illness narratives and participate in the community. If the women were rigid in their structure, diction, and conversation and based their evaluation of members' credibility on writing structure, the space would be demanding and members would not feel the freedom to freely, transparently, and authentically discourse. Authenticity brings the community together—they need not share the level of expertise in writing or researching or even in their knowledge of their disease; they need only be participants of the community, accepted because they share the same fate of a diagnosis of breast cancer and they are willing to *share.*

The rhetoric of breast cancer is based on discourse by the patients who are experiencing and confronting the disease. Therefore, the discourse reflects them—their purposes, their emotions, their knowledge of writing (as the discussion board is text based), and their communication styles. The rhetoric of breast cancer also contains content related to the members' *logos*, *ethos*, and *pathos* as the members seek to interact. The content also relates to the members' efforts to persuade other members.

LOGOS, ETHOS, AND *PATHOS*

Although Aristotle identifies three appeals or proofs that serve as the rhetor's rhetorical strategy, strategy requires planning and critical thinking. The rhetor (speaker, writer, poster . . .) anticipates the audience's response and applies *logos*, *ethos*, and *pathos*. Within the discourse on Breastcancer.org's discussion board, the community members may not strategize on their communication—they may not think of the impact their posts will have—as much as they seek to honestly and authentically communicate as part of the community. However, the appeals of *logos*, *ethos*, and *pathos* are evident within the discourse.

Logical appeals (*logos*) are present in the discourse with these illness narratives. Illness narratives are full of arguments, statements, and processes that are supported by data and facts. The facts include the medical evidence surrounding the patients' diagnoses as well as resources that healthcare professionals provide (and they provide each patient diagnosed with breast cancer with a huge bag of resources) and resources that patients have found for themselves. Their illness narratives are also full of facts about the women's experiences with the disease. But the illness narrative also involves how the patient feels, how much the medical care costs, the effects on the patient's family, the side effects from the disease and the treatments, and many other facts that are evidence of the patient's disease and treatment—and of her humanity. Patients will make arguments about struggles and also about parts of the treatments that they do not like, and they support those arguments with cited evidence from elements of their narratives.

Ethical appeals (*ethos*) within the disease narrative are based on the woman's experience with the disease—has she been diagnosed and is her disease narrative believable—and also by the woman's character, most frequently evident in the community by how a community member treats other members. But the women also build their *ethos* by sharing resources and citing their sources, not with formal citation styles but with information that verifies the credibility of the resource and the woman's presentation of it (e.g., where she found the resource or what she learned from it). Identity is an important part of the appeals in this community; in fact, the administration of Breastcancer.org requires *ethos* by requiring that members register to establish their identity within the online community and by removing posts that do not align with the purpose of the discussion board (as shared in chapter 1).

The appeal of *pathos* is the easiest and most obvious appeal in the discourse within the discussion board of Breastcancer.org. The purpose of Breastcancer.org is to provide an informative and safe online community for patients who have been diagnosed with a frequent and sometimes terminal disease, a diagnosis that can bring fear, anger, confusion, appreciation, joy, and sympathy. The emotions related to the disease are an anticipated part of the illness narratives that women share in their posts. However, the emotions are not limited to the patients who are posting; within their narratives, they also share how their families and friends are dealing with their diagnoses. The *pathos* is also extreme: in some posts, the women express their value of life and love, and in other posts, they express their fear, particularly of the unknowns related to their disease processes. (I will address these emotional appeals later in this chapter.)

As stated in the introduction, rhetoric is a cooperative act in which the members are acting together (Segal, 2005, p. 12). These members are acting together, applying *logos*, *ethos*, and *pathos* to relate to each other—to understand and believe the arguments that they share, to build their credibility within the community and discourse with identity, and to share the emotional elements of their illness narratives that makes them share their humanity. In coding the discourse in the threads from Breastcancer.org, I recognized the action of the community members and thus frequently coded with notations such as "expressing agency," "sharing experience," "asking questions," or "commenting on care." (In this way, I differed from coding schemes used by Blank and Adams-Blodnieks [2007] and Radin [2006], who focused on categories of post content, like "a query" or "information." This allowed me to also note action and rhetorical elements.)

PERSUASION

Traditionally, the art of rhetoric focused on the persuasive elements of the communication being analyzed. Persuasiveness is a quality that is part of the discourse taking place within a medically focused discussion board and specifically on Breastcancer.org: the women who are posting are seeking to interact and thus need to persuade the other members that they belong in the community and thus should be included in the discourse. In seeking to persuade, a member who posts is seeking to "[make her] view of things compelling" (Lyne, 2001, p. 3) to the other members, with *compelling* meaning "tending to compel, as to force or push toward a course of action . . . having a powerful and irresistible effect; requiring acute admiration, attention, or respect" ("compelling," n.d.). She is then seeking to share her experiences through her illness narrative and thus compelling other members to include and interact with her. The purpose is not to have others directly state, "You compel me" but to participate and interact—establishing *logos*, *ethos*, and *pathos* so that members respond positively. (Members can respond negatively, although I only witnessed that one time in 676 posts with a reference of thanks because the administration of Breastcancer.org removed an inappropriate post. This incidence is addressed in chapter 1.)

An additional purpose of the persuasive elements is to share hope: "The preacher uses rhetoric to give the audience hope. Much of contemporary rhetoric, even practical and political rhetoric, revolves around the interpretation of texts in a way whose importance and complications are not adequately covered by Aristotle's remarks about the *atechnoi* of judicial rhetoric" (Garver, 2009, p. 6). Hope is one of those purposes that does not fit into *atechnoi*; hope depends on anticipation but is not necessarily grounded in evidence. In this way, Garver is correct: hope is not covered by Aristotle's standards. Hope requires an optimistic expectation: individual anticipates that a situation's outcome will be positive—a necessity in the rhetoric related to any disease because the patient hopes that the diagnosis is correct, that the treatment is going to succeed, that the outcome will be a cure and a better life, and that the recovery will be complete. Therefore, online communities—where individuals can interact with others who "speak their language"—provide valuable resources for patients who need hope. In those communities, they are not patients as much as they are individuals who have a disease and are going to go through a treatment to (they hope) eliminate the disease from their body, having survived the influence that the disease has on their lives in the interim as well as being able to return to some normalcy. They can seek others who speak the same rhetoric, they can interject medical terminology related to their illness narratives, and together, members can apply the rhetoric of their disease (including those medical terms) to gain hope. Together. Hope is a valuable outcome in rhetoric, including in the rhetoric of breast cancer.

ACCURACY OF REPORTED CONTENT

Whereas some online communities exist for members to voice their opinions and preferences, Breastcancer.org exists because the members share a medical diagnosis. A large majority of the members in this online community are not healthcare providers; a few of the members note that they are medical staff, but they too are battling breast cancer and thus are qualified and accepted members of the community. As a result of the nonmedical population in the community, the shared information comes from other resources—typically from members' research, medical charts, and conversations with their healthcare providers—and thus comes through a filter of non-medically trained individuals. This information cannot be verified for accuracy.

Individuals who join these online communities seek to exchange information (Eastin, 2001; Krcmar and Leimeister, 2005; Orgad, 2005; Sharf, 1997). They may be aware that not all information online is accurate (Biermann, Golladay, Greenfield, and Baker, 1999; Borzekowski, Schenk, Wilson, and Peebles, 2010; Eastin, 2001; Huang and Penson, 2008; Jones, 2009; Lissman and Boehnlein, 2001; Still, 2008), and inaccuracies can be life-threatening for those who act on incorrect information; therefore, they must carefully discern which information about treatments they will accept, consume, and follow. As stated earlier, patients are using the World Wide Web more frequently for health-related information, but they are guarded about the information they find online (Huang and Penson, 2008). Physicians too are guarded about patients using the Internet for medical information (Huang and Penson, 2008; Kim and Kim, 2009; Tann, Platts, Welch, and Allen, 2003; Zun, Blume, Lester, Simpson, and Downey, 2004; Zun, Downey, and Brown, 2011), expressing concern because the reading levels of medical information are too complex for many patients to understand, because patients expect unrealistic outcomes as a result of the information they read online, and because quality information is not accessible to patients (Huang and Penson, 2008). (The standards for "quality" also are not consistent.) This concern about accuracy has fueled research as well as an objective in *Healthy People 2020* (2017), which established a goal for accurate information online. Patient and provider concerns come from research that focuses on the World Wide Web but rarely evaluates the content within communities of individuals who are undergoing treatments.

In online communities, anyone who can access the Internet can post; therefore, those who seek information on the Internet must be careful to note who is posting (American Cancer Society, 2016; Huang and Penson 2008). "Studies have often been concerned with aspects of the verifiability, credibility, trustworthiness and accuracy of the information on these [health-related] sites" (Orgad, 2005, p. 2–3), particularly because more and more, people are using these communities as sources of information about health and medicine (Bunde, Suis, Martin, and Barnett, 2006; Cline and Haynes, 2001; Finfgeld, 2000; Whitten, Smith, Munday, and LaPlante, 2008). Inaccurate information, that can include inaccurate language, can be a liability for those who access and act on it, and current research shows that "[1] in 20 breast cancer Web pages featured inaccuracies, and sites displaying complementary and alternative medicine were 15 times more likely to contain false or misleading health information" (Cahill, 2008, para. 1).

The designers and administrators of online communities are concerned about accuracy and even the resulting liability related to inaccurate information. For example, WebMD Communities posts a disclaimer to remind the community members that accuracy may be an issue:

> The opinions expressed in WebMD Communities are solely those of the User, who may or may not have medical or scientific training. These opinions do not represent the opinions of WebMD. Communities are not reviewed by a WebMD physician or any member of the WebMD editorial staff for accuracy, balance, objectivity, or any other reason except for compliance with our Terms and Conditions. Some of these opinions may contain information about treatments or uses of drug products that have not been approved by the U.S. Food and Drug Administration. WebMD does not endorse any specific product, service or treatment.
>
> Do not consider Communities as medical advice. Never delay or disregard seeking professional medical advice from your doctor or other qualified healthcare provider because of something you have read on WebMD. You should always speak with your doctor before you start, stop, or change any prescribed part of your care plan or treatment. WebMD understands that reading individual, real-life experiences can be a helpful resource, but it is never a substitute for professional medical advice, diagnosis, or treatment from a qualified health care provider. If you think you may have a medical emergency, call your doctor or dial 911 immediately. (WebMD LLC, 2016)

The American Cancer Society (2016) has posted a similar disclaimer, formatted as a warning to individuals who use any Website for information about cancer:

> Cancer information on the Internet comes from many different sources—expert health organizations, government agencies, universities, merchants, interest groups, the general public, and scam artists. Anyone can post any kind of information online and some people may be passing along information that's limited, inaccurate, or just plain wrong. Some even try to deceive you.
>
> Scam artists and other dishonest people use the Internet for 2 main reasons: low cost and relative anonymity (no one knows who they are). What's more, the message or product gets out to people all over the world.
>
> The nature of the web makes it easier to mislead people. For example, if you saw a sign in front of a small, run-down store that claimed it was the largest supplier of medical devices in the United States, you'd probably be suspicious right away. But if you saw a professional-looking website making the same claim, you might have a harder time deciding if it was real.
>
> This is not to say that you shouldn't trust anything on the Internet—just that you have to choose your sources carefully. Even on trusted, highly regarded websites, it's important to note that the health information is just general information that might not apply to you at all. *Always remember that information found online should not take the place of medical advice.* If you have a health-related problem, please talk to a doctor. There's no other way to get the same experience and care as sitting down with a health care provider who can

> look at your health history, your unique medical situation, examine you, and talk with you about how you've been feeling.

The warning of false or inaccurate information is valid; individuals may invade an online community and post false information or present a false identity to disrupt the discourse—for reasons such as gratification, power, or revenge. Other members of the community will seek to share their experiences but may inadvertently misquote a physician or source or simply share inaccurate information because they are not medical experts.

Accurate information is important and the evidence that members share is important. However, accuracy is not required in the rhetoric of breast cancer. Members do not filter information to ensure its accuracy; however, they do apply the rhetorical appeals to measure the information they are gathering. They can consider the *pathos* that the member presents (e.g., Why was she searching information and how does she respond and relate to the information and to other members?); they can consider the *ethos* of the member presenting the information (e.g., Has she presented believable and evidence-based information?); and they can consider the *logos* of the evidence that a member presents (e.g., Does she provide credible resources and does her argument make sense, compared to what I know and what my healthcare provider has told me?). In this way, because the members of this online community are interacting, they seem to self-regulate the online community and thus research to verify the data that other members share. The members may not catch inaccurate information, but if one member posts a question, another member shares information to answer that question, citing her sources, and then other members can agree, ask further questions to try the first answer, or offer alternative answers.

CUSTOMIZED RHETORIC

Most diseases are referenced with customized rhetoric—terms and explanations that are specific to the symptoms and the organisms (e.g., bacteria, viruses, irregular DNA) related to the disease; the tests that expose the evidence of the disease; the specialists who are trained to recognize and treat the disease; the illness (such as lifestyle influences) that the disease brings; the treatments and side effects related to treatment; and the patients who carry the disease and experience the illness.

Language in particular is an important part of health and medical communication. Patients may seek information, but because healthcare providers have their own culture (Charles, Gafni, and Whelan, 2000), patients may not connect via medical rhetoric (the general rhetoric of the medical community) with their providers. Patients may not "speak" the same language as healthcare specialists and may not have training in physiology to understand the disease process. They may not know how to ask questions, and they may be overwhelmed in the medical environment and with the circumstances of their diseases (Bellwoar, 2012, p. 327). They may not understand the medical terminology related to surgery, oncology, radiology, and other fields of medicine or have any idea what to question. Patients go into a medical appointment seeking information about prevention, diagnoses, and treatment and leave overwhelmed and unsure of what is going on in their own bodies. As they go through the experience of breast cancer, they begin to pick up the language that relates to their own narratives. But they may never speak the medical jargon that their physicians and providers speak.

Breast cancer has its own vocabulary. Terms like "mastectomy," "BRCA1" and "BRCA2," "DIEP tissue flap," "fine needle aspiration," "chemotherapy," and "WBCs" begin to take on meaning after an individual hears, "You have breast cancer." But the language goes further than the name of the disease: patients learn their stages, grades, and types of breast cancer. They learn about the treatments they will undergo—standards for cancer practice that involve biopsies, surgical procedures, chemotherapy with certain drugs, radiation, and possible reconstruction. Patients learn how their bodies work and how cancer, surgery, chemotherapy, radiation, and other processes affect their bodies, and they use specific and technical terms to inform and persuade with information related to their diagnoses. They see the facial expressions from each other and from their providers and caregivers, they feel the symptoms and side effects, they hear the discussions, and they overhear nonverbal communication with the sounds of technology and providers. As part of their experience with breast cancer, they use the rhetoric of breast cancer.

The rhetoric of breast cancer includes a shared action, which is necessary for members to persuade each other to commune, discourse, cooperatively act, share, and hope. Healthcare providers, communicators, patient advocates, and other professionals who work in the medical field understand medical rhetoric and use medical terminology—the language of their experience, training, and profession (Barton, 2004). Their language relates to the complex language that they as trained professionals have learned to effectively communicate within the medical community. However, these professionals speak medical rhetoric; they need to consider how individuals diagnosed with breast cancer use cancer-related language and culture to interact about their disease.

As patients communicate with each other, they learn, create, and adopt terms related to their illnesses so they can express their emotions and struggles. Patients do not need to learn medical rhetoric; they need only the language related to their disease. With that rhetoric, the patients "share information, express their feelings and offer support" (Orgad, 2005, p. 16). They share information about their diagnoses and treatments as well as their opinions of their healthcare providers. These patients share the resources that they have found as they have researched their diagnoses; the emotions that they are experiencing through illness; the logistical problems (finances, insurance, and appointments) that they face; and other information that reflects the values and rhetorics of the community. These patients use the language related to their medical diagnoses and treatment. And the members of Breastcancer.org use and expand the rhetoric of breast cancer.

RHETORICAL ANALYSIS OF BREASTCANCER.ORG POSTS

The members posting in the discussion board of Breastcancer.org discuss a variety of topics; this analysis addresses their discussions on resources related to breast cancer, on their emotions (specifically fear and gratitude), on their struggles with finances and with the "waiting" related to their treatments, and on their names for their diseases. Many of these members integrate these themes into their use of the rhetoric of breast cancer, and other members agree and add to the discourse.

Resources

The members of Breastcancer.org share a variety of resources—articles, videos, books, and other sources that they find during their research and that they think other community members might need or want. Other studies of online communities (Bunde, Suis, Martin, and Barnett, 2006; Cline and Haynes, 2001; Finfgeld, 2000; Whitten, Smith, Munday, and LaPlante, 2008) have found that this is typical. Shared resources create a rich source of information for members in the online community. The types of resources differ, depending on the purpose of the thread. However, they all relate to breast cancer—to prevention, diagnosis, treatment, or recovery—and they all apply the rhetoric of breast cancer.

Different circumstances encourage different rhetorical elements—such as differing tones, purposes, and terms. For example, women discussing medical and alternative healthcare options in the Breastcancer.org thread "Progesterone Cream" seek to learn how to monitor and replace changing hormones, and they share sources of information related to and thus including language related to hormone levels and replacement. (Some breast cancers are fueled by estrogen and progesterone—hormones that the body naturally makes—so hormone levels, including levels affected by the natural process of menopause, may be a consideration because of the type of disease.) These women recommend books related to the topic for the thread of posts—particularly related to hormones—including *Estrogen: How is it Bad for You* and *Hormone Heresy*. They post links and reviews for informative Websites other than Breastcancer.org, such as kokorohealth.com and womentowomen.com.

They share information obtained from resources on television and YouTube as well as articles from medical journals like *Current Cancer Drug Targets*, *Journal of the National Cancer Institute*, and *International Journal of Cancer*. One member shares an email from Marisa Weiss, MD, the founder of Breastcancer.org; the email is a response to questions that the woman sends to Dr. Weiss. In this thread in the online community, the women share resources that they gather, most often from healthcare providers and researchers; these resources are evidence based. In providing these sources, they provide the names of the sources and they sometimes add the Web address to build their credibility and the *ethos* of the sources they are sharing.

On Breastcancer.org, while the thread "Progesterone Cream" addresses holistic treatments related to hormone imbalances, the threads "MPBC" and "Just Diagnosed" exist for different purposes. The thread "MPBC" involves the discourse of only six women, but their language is targeted because they share a diagnosis—metaplastic breast cancer. This type of breast cancer is rare and the population with metaplastic breast cancer is small. Early in the members' conversation, one member states that another thread of posts focusing on metaplastic breast cancer exists on Breastcancer.org, and the members discuss moving their conversation from the present thread to the other to unify the conversation and thus merge their discourse. Although they do not post references to online and print resources, as do the members in the "Progesterone Cream" thread, the members on "MPBC" recognize the threads of posts about the members' disease as well as their discourse as credible resources. They also recognize that another group of members with metaplastic breast cancer "speak their language" and relate to the specific details and experiences that patients with this diagnosis experience. This subpopulation of Breastcancer.org shows that online community members sometimes "cluster" depending on their diagnoses—so they can more specifically discuss their disease (a type of breast cancer) and communicate within the culture (the language, the experiences, the specific struggles) of their particular diagnosis. Their rhetoric is specialized per their diagnoses. And, by suggesting that they merge threads to merge the sub-communities of women with metaplastic breast cancer (MPBC), these members establish their *pathos*, their understanding that the other members are weary and busy and do not need additional sites to visit; their *logos*, that perhaps they should merge with another thread to unify the conversation related to these members' specific breast-cancer diagnosis; and their *ethos* by being open to options that are best for the community members.

In contrast, the thread "Just Diagnosed" starts as a place where newly diagnosed community members can find basic introductory resources. However, new members begin to post their introductions in this thread and the discourse expands. New members introduce themselves, seeking to join the community and establish their *ethos* as members; they do not share only their usernames and locations, but they also share their diagnoses in detail, expanding their rhetoric to build *ethos* as breast-cancer patients. In response, older members respond with encouragement and resources to answer the new members' concerns. These resources include

- online resources other than Breastcancer.org (17 references),
- other threads on Breastcancer.org (12 referenccs),
- print resources–books and pamphlets (7 references), and
- organizations and agencies that offer information and services (4 references).

By sharing these resources and seeking to give new members hope, "older" members respond with a tone that resonates *pathos*—"We are here, and we understand."—and *ethos*—"You can ask questions here, and you can find additional help with these resources." (As the source of these resources, the older members build their credibility with the new members.)

As detailed earlier, accuracy of the information shared in online communities is a concern because anyone who registers as part of the community can share information in the discussion boards and chat rooms. Inaccurate information is potentially available on Webpages that are not created and maintained by credentialed entities. However, members on Breastcancer.org seek to provide accurate information by "citing" their sources: not in a standard citation format (such as the American Psychological Association style or the American Medical Association style, which would be appropriate for the content of their resources), but by providing enough information that other members can find these resources. (If other members cannot find the resources, they can return to the discourse and ask for additional information about where a resource exists.)

By sharing resources, members build their credibility, their *ethos*, and that of the community of Breastcancer.org by establishing the online community as a source of information for patients with breast cancer. (Logic tells us that the members of this community come to gather accurate information.) In the community, women who share multiple sources of evidence build their *ethos* and those who share their illness narratives build their *pathos.* This *ethos* and *pathos* is recognized when one member (Brenna) acknowledges her faith in the credibility of the community members by posting,

> It's one thing [information] coming from doctors its totally different coming from a real person who has went through it.

(I will offer more examples of this in the other sections in this chapter.)

By sharing their experiences and using credible sources and relevant language, the members also build the *ethos* of Breastcancer.org as a credible source. For example, the justification page for the "Just Diagnosed" thread (started by Paula) states,

> This may be a helpful pace to begin to reading to get the facts in order, and know how to move through each step as well as coping with the fear of diagnoses.
>
> - www.Breastcancer.org/cmn_copi_fear_diag.html
> - www.Breastcancer.org/dia_pict_idx.html"[1]

The member who created the initial post of the "Just Diagnosed" thread identifies Breastcancer.org (and two pages in particular) as a credible starting place for newly diagnosed members who are seeking information. The members acknowledge this and the credibility of the virtual space: one active member (Virginia) who has posted 3,291 posts on Breastcancer.org, states, "This is also one of the best places I have found to get information about breast cancer, its treatments, and living with the disease." Another member (Ashlynn), who works in the medical field, posts that Breastcancer.org is a source for "correct information." As noted earlier, accuracy is a concern, and with thousands of members, the online community will have inaccurate information. But the community members believe that overall the community is a valuable, accurate, and credible source. In this way, new members are persuaded to return to the online community to gather information because they can trust that the members are seeking to share accurate information.

Emotion

In addition to sharing resources, women within this community share what they are feeling, thus building their *pathos* as fellow humans and patients who potentially are experiencing the same emotions as other members within the community. The members seek to express those emotions with words and in ways that other members can relate; members are allowed (even encouraged) to express their emotions by others who ask and who openly share their own feelings. A patient's family members can sympathize, but if they have not gone through the disease process and thus experienced the feelings that go with that disease, they cannot fully relate. In contrast, community members who are going through the same experience can draw near to a woman who is newly diagnosed with breast cancer and they can empathetically share the experience by sharing their own feelings. This sharing builds a strong *pathos* within the community because members express understanding and care.

The medical diagnosis of breast cancer potentially creates diverse emotions within the patient. The individual facing the diagnosis may not be prepared to understand the repercussions of the diagnosis and may experience a broad spectrum of emotions. She may hear the diagnosis and need time to think about what questions she has and what feelings she experiences. The first emotion is usually fear—fear of the unknown—although a patient's fear may decrease as she moves through the disease process and knows more about what to expect from day to day.

In Breastcancer.org, community members share the spectrum of emotions that they experience during the process of their disease: from when they hear "You have breast cancer" and face having cancer (a sometimes-terminal disease), to facing radiation or chemotherapy, to undergoing an amputation, and to finally receiving report of remission or full healing from breast cancer. Breast cancer is a particularly difficult diagnosis: it has a public "face," intimate nature, difficult treatments, and sometimes morbid outcome. Even with remission, a patient usually loses her breast, an organ that is a visual part of her identity as a woman, and must live with a missing breast or, if she undergoes reconstruction, a recreated breast that is void of the neurological (nerve) connections that give a woman breast sensitivity. Facing these possibilities can be overwhelming.

Expressing emotion is beneficial to patients, as proven by research (e.g., Beaudoin and Tao, 2007; Pennebaker, 1990; Pennebaker, 1993; Rodgers and Chen, 2005; and addressed in the introduction). Thus, the rhetoric of breast cancer also includes language and expression of patients' feelings about the disease and a shared *pathos* within the community. In particular, members of Breastcancer.org express negative emotions that include fear, confusion, frustration, anger, hopelessness, and overwhelmed-ness and positive emotions that include happiness and relief. For example, in the "MPBC" thread, in thirty-one posts, these six women referenced fifty-three emotions, including

- thanks, appreciation, gratitude, and gladness (for others, their information, or the thread);
- regret;
- unspecified negative feelings;
- fear; and
- unspecified positive feelings.

They express gratitude most often, using different terms for these feelings of gratitude that are embedded within their narrative. Similarly, in the 176 posts of the "Just Diagnosed" thread, members included 212 references to emotions, including

- fear,
- appreciation and thanks for others and for life,
- uncertainty and feelings about the unknown,

- shock,
- optimism or positive feelings,
- a desire to stay positive,
- confusion,
- worry,
- hope, and
- overwhelmed-ness.

New members introducing themselves and sharing their initial surge of feelings express that, in addition to these emotions, they feel numb, concerned, depressed, and frustrated. Members who share feelings of fear tend to express their agency, talking about what frightens them and how they want to respond. In response, other members encourage them to cope with their fear; they connect through *pathos* and encourage the new members to hope for the best. Members who use words of gratitude express appreciation for a variety of people and circumstances—feelings that seem to relate directly with the members' attitudes about their diagnoses.

The two emotions that are most frequent and most important in the discourse between members are fear and gratitude (or appreciation). The following sections discuss the community members' expressions of these feelings, quoting their statements to allow their voices and the *pathos* expressed in the rhetoric of breast cancer to be prominent.

Fear

Many people experience fear when they first receive their diagnosis of cancer (Ashing-Giwa and Lim, 2010; Ballard-Reisch and Letner, 2003; Gill and Babrow, 2007; Gremore, Baucom, Porter, et al., 2011; Morgan, 2009; Tiedtke, de Rijk, de Casterle, Christiaens, and Donceel, 2010). They experience fear because the word "cancer" brings the unknown and they are unsure of the outcome of their disease; they may expect to experience a negative outcome if they know someone who previously confronted breast cancer. When women diagnosed with breast cancer enter a community where they can openly discuss their disease experience, they have the freedom to express that fear. Just as the members differ, their fears and how they express fear differ, and their responses to fear illustrate how the members of the community interact and share their narratives. But the important element is that the members empathize and encourage each other to face those fears.

Within the discourse of Breastcancer.org, some members identify what they fear and others simply state that they are afraid. Regardless of if they know what they fear, their fear is a part of the rhetoric of breast cancer and is regularly present in the discourse in the discussion board. In the thread titled "Progesterone Cream," only six members express fear—perhaps the lowest rate of references to number of participants because a majority of the women posting in this thread speak in past tense. Therefore, they have completed their treatments for breast cancer and now focus on recovery, particularly the symptoms in their recovery that relate to altered hormone levels resulting from breast cancer treatment. These women have faced the unknown of the disease process and are now returning to some sense of normalcy in their lives. Then, they relate their feelings to hormone imbalances and empathize as they share that part of the experience.

In the thread titled "MPBC," one member (Katie) references fear four times, stating that the diagnosis of breast cancer is scary and also that her physician warns her not to research too much and become frightened:

> I agree w/ [another member]—it's therapeutic and a release for my jumbled and rather frightened mind about all this. . . . basically saying' they didn't know what to make of it . . . a little frightening, huh!
>
> . . . when she [surgeon] called me with the results she said, 'now don't go out there online and start reading about this because it will literally scare u out of your mind. . . . i proceeded to read, read, read and finally decided that it was too overwhelming and too scarey.

The analysis of this post cannot overlook the informality of Katie's post: among other mechanics and style issues, she uses text-type abbreviations for "with" and "you," she does not capitalize "I," and she misspells "scarey." However, the formality of her message or the mechanical correctness of her post is not the rhetoric focus, although her comfort level is important. What does matter is that the message of her post is clearly expressed; she researches, even after her surgeon tells her not to, and she realizes that the information is scaring and overwhelming her. She shares her experience with a group of women who are not newly diagnosed; they are well into the treatment stages of their disease processes and, therefore, have experienced what Katie is experiencing. Katie, who is the most recently diagnosed member of this group of six women, feels the freedom to share her emotions because the other members then have established their credibility and their empathy as fellow breast-cancer patients and she knows they understand.

In the thread titled "Just Diagnosed," numerous members share that they are experiencing fear. Paula starts the thread by mentioning "the fear of diagnosis," and Kat, empathizing, responds:

> Needless to say, I'm scared. I can't imagine anyone wouldn't be getting that kind of information [a diagnosis of breast cancer].

Members respond to each other's specific fears, such as this connection per the members' fears about diagnosis. In this way, they express *pathos* and connect.

Other members express that they fear the outcome of their diagnoses. For example, Gail shares, "[I am] scared for my outcome, I just feel like I have a few positive things but more negative," and Winnie shares

> I fear the outcome. I don't know how I am going to get thru the next 3 weeks, and this is just the beginning. I just read through the forum and cried. So many emotions.

Nina expresses similar fear:

> Family and friends have been very supportive, but they don't have the answers. I never realized how much control you need to take when dealing with breast cancer. So many decisions to make, and very scary because they are about your survival.

In this way, these women realize that fellow breast-cancer patients may have answers and the online community's discussion board is a safe place to share a fear that many other members are expressing. And, as Nina expresses, they feel each other's emotions, particularly their fears. They share those fears.

One member, Margaret, relates her fear to her experiences in school during the Nuclear Age:

> I had never been an outwardly emotional person but found myself crying everywhere I went: at work and with friends and family. I was terrified of chemo and had always had a fear of radiation. I think that was from the duck and cover school days of the 1950's.

While other members in the community may not be old enough to relate to the presented parallel of cancer treatment to the fear of nuclear bombs, they do relate to the fear of radiation—the unknowns of burning the cancer with radiation treatments.

Fear goes beyond the women who are diagnosed with breast cancer, and community members may be aware of their family members' fears about the diagnosis and treatments. For example, Sandra shares, "My husband is fearful of wating another 4 weeks before we get this thing out of me and start treatment." Sandra does not share that she is experiencing fear, but she relates her husband's fearful feelings about her diagnosis. In that way, she acknowledges her husband's fear, not diminishing it but building her own *pathos* by caring that her husband is afraid and by sharing that with the other members of the community.

Community members may fear that they will not be able to perform everyday tasks and that their inability to function with excellence may affect others. One particularly detailed post from Sharon, a school teacher, provides insight into her feelings and concerns about how her diagnosis will affect her students and her work. Sharon writes,

> I've just been diagnosed . . . and my worst fear is leaving my 130+ middle school language arts kids in the hands of a long term sub, or worse numerous subs if they can't find a long term sub to cover the whole time, in my absence. . . . I fear chemo will weaken my immune system and being exposed to all the illnesses schools inherently have would be a bad thing. Also, having so many essays to correct . . . and hearing fatigues and foggy thinking etc makes me stressed all ready. How will I do it?

Sharon's concern relates to her students and how her disease will affect them as well as her ability to complete every-day tasks that her job requires. She shares her fear with an empathetic community and also expresses her care about her students, which builds her *pathos* and *ethos* with the other members because, rather than fearing how she will handle the cancer, she fears that she cannot fully serve her students.

Another source of fear is the unknown of breast cancer, either because the women do not know what is going on or because they read what may happen and they are frightened by what they read. Several members share this fear in the thread for newly diagnosed members:

- Gayle: "I am so scared because i don't know what is going on."
- Konstanze (representing her mother): "The more information, and understanding, will help give her knowledge [and] might reduce her fears."
- Susan: "I am frightened and depressed. I feel almost afraid to ask questions about my breast cancer."
- Deborah: "I've done a lot of research which has helped but also terrifies me."

Similarly, Whitney writes, "I know reading stuff online has been frightening to me. Maybe I should wait to research after I know more [about my diagnosis]." In response to Whitney, Adrian (an active member with 8,248 posts) responds,

> RE: research, please limit your research to sites like this or other valid ones, and yes, wait till you have some good info about YOUR pathology before overloading yourself with information that will certainly keep you up nights!

And Shari agrees: "Adrian is right . . . try not to scare yourself by doing research until you know YOUR specifics. . . . I did that and scared the living daylights out of myself." Then Kristy responds, seeking to encourage these women:

> Many of us are petrified when diagnosed and even beyond. I fell into the category of "knowledge is power", as it took my fear, and, with my doctors, helped move my thoughts into an action plan and hope.

And Bridgett agrees: "You've come to the right place to get info. Understanding your treatment will help you deal with the fear of the unknown." In this particular interaction between members, the *pathos* that exists within the rhetoric of breast cancer is particularly evident: newly diagnosed women openly express their fears, and members who are further along in the disease process and who have faced the same fears build their *ethos* and *pathos* by affirming these newer members. They share the new members' fears and also advise them on how to alleviate their fears—to wait to research until the members know their diagnoses, to learn from their healthcare providers and from members within Breastcancer.org and other credible communities, and to focus on hope.

The rhetoric of breast cancer does not require that women who are experiencing breast cancer feel the same fear, and members in this online community acknowledge that their fears may differ. Cathy expresses this idea well in one of her posts:

> There are some special concerns and fears for those of us not diagnosed at earlier stages, but you will find many of us on that thread [another thread for patients diagnosed at stage 3 breast cancer] that have finished treatment and feel great, positive and very optimistic.

That interaction, focused on empathy, is evident when Deanna posts her introduction—"Scared to death. I came here to find people in my same board."—and Brigid also introduces herself, relating to the community that will understand:

> I am so scared. My family and friends have been extremely supportive but I thought I would join here for more support. . . . I really can't believe this is happening to me. I am sure you are all aware how shocking it is and that we share the same feelings and fears.

In this community, empathy (shared *pathos*) is an important and consistent response to other members' fears, be they about the disease, the unknown, the side effects of treatment, or some other complication that the disease process creates. Fear is shared, and members can express their fear without being concerned that the other members will shun their feelings. The interaction and shared feelings further build the sense of community in Breastcancer.org and strengthens the shared rhetoric of breast cancer.

Ironically, in the face of fear of this unknown, inconsistent, and sometimes terminal disease, members discourse and the rhetoric of breast cancer rarely include a reference to the members' fear of death or mortality. Members may use trite sayings such as "scared to death," and one member (Gracie) jokingly states,

> I've researched this MBC [metaplastic breast cancer] triple negative BC [breast cancer] to death (pardon the expression). I just felt I needed more information. (I'm a research junkie.).

However, conversation related to death typically has two themes: first, that someone else has died or second, that members are assuring new members that they are not going to die because of breast cancer. This is, then, an example of community members using persuasive language to encourage other members to feel hope, although they cannot predict another members' outcome.

First, community members share with each other about family members who have died. They talk about how the death fits into their disease process, thus placing it in context and addressing how difficult it is to lose a family member during the challenges of breast cancer. For example, Lydia writes,

> Tonight my husband and I took a bike ride to the cemetary where we will be placing my mom this week. . . . it's really very beautiful and peaceful there, and I will be glad to have somewhere so close to go visit her. She actually died in Feb of 0000,[2] was cremated, and it took us some time to figure out what to do since she didn't specify. I had just started chemo when she died, it was soooo hard, she was my best friend, and just one of a kind ☺.

In response, Katie shares about her own loss:

> I lost my dad last summer and he is buried in another state. Thank goodness, he didn't have to see me go thru this. i was his 'little girl' and it would have brought on major medical issues for him if this had occurred when he was still alive.

Lydia then responds to Katie with sympathy:

> I'm sorry about your dad, it is hard to deal with losing a parent. I know what you mean, I felt terrible that my mom was sick, but worrying about me at the same time; I actually felt partially responsible for her dying at first, thinking it stressed her too much. Of course I know that isn't what happened now.

And another established community member, Michele, greets a new member acknowledging that the women share about losing family members:

> Welcome! I'm sorry you have to join us here, but we're glad to have you. I've read your story, and in so many ways it is similar to what all of us on this thread have experienced . . . even the death of a loved one during dg/tx

> [diagnosis/treatment]. Two of the other ladies lost parents at about the same time in their journey as you did. How terribly difficult that must have been.

In the "Newly Diagnosed" thread, two women (Lorraine and Bekah) reference their family members who recently died. They share how they have lost family members during the disease process and thus express and experience empathy in a different theme of their discourse. In this discourse, members share that they have needed to cope with loss while they are undergoing treatment. Other members express empathy—that others have lost family members during the disease process—and in that way share the grief. Unexpectedly, the community members do not relate others' deaths to their own mortality.

Second, in the rhetoric of breast cancer, death is referenced and dismissed as community members respond that breast cancer does not result in death. In fact, references to death are notably absent or are contained within the discourse (Orgad, 2005, p. 176). The most frequently references occur in the "Just Diagnosed" thread, where women who have recently learned that they have breast cancer are introducing themselves. Their comments less frequently express fear of death and more frequently acknowledge that they know they will not die from breast cancer:

- Margaret: "When I was diagnosed . . . I was petrified and was sure I was going to die." (Margaret uses past tense because she *was* sure, but she has more information now and understands that, depending on the stage, grade, and type of cancer, she will survive.)
- Amy: "[M]y husband said I'm not going anyplace until we pay the medical bills off. His way of saying that I will be here for a long time." and "[T]hese message boards give me so much hope and strength reading all of your stories, now I know that breast cancer isn't a death sentence. Thank all of you ladies for posting."
- Lesley: "My life is over isn't it?? I feel like I have just been handed my death sentence."

Even Lesley's question is framed in a question and a feeling rather than a reality; these members address their fears in the past or with reference to a "death sentence," which is an inappropriate metaphor because these women have not committed crimes and thus are not being punished (or sentenced).

The sense of *logos*, *ethos*, and *pathos* is evident in the experienced members' responses. They assure new members that life does not end when they are diagnosed with breast cancer. They relate to new members' concerns but explain, as experienced members of the community and women who have already gone through part of the disease process, that these women will not die of breast cancer. Using the rhetoric of breast cancer, these experienced members address new members' concerns:

- Paige: "Don't get all worked up over your pathology report and don't think this is an automatic death sentence because it isn't."
- Margaret: "The reality is/was . . . I haven't died and won't for a very long time."
- Sharon: "It is awful. I know it is, but really there is so much hope for cancer patients these days. The survival rate is great, although the process sucks for sure . . . it really is all going to be OK. Cancer is not a death sentence anymore."

These women defy death in their responses, sharing with others that they are not going to die. Other members expand their assurances; Janie posts:

> All of this is beyond overwhelming, but by NO means is it a death sentence. There are people on this board that were actually told it was a death sentence and are still kicking. There are new treatments being found every day. Like the saying goes "This isn't your mama's cancer". That is so true. My mom died of cancer 14 yrs. Ago. If they had the treatments then that they have today I believe she would still be with us. That is why I know that I will be around for my kids.

And Hayley adds a little subtle humor to her response:

> Take a deep breath (there's always time to worry later . . .). . . . I've seen survival rates noted at 99%+ for five years . . . and suggestions that the ones who died were "hit by the bus on the way to the hospital." Nothing to do w/ [with] the BC [breast cancer].

These women build their logos by acknowledging that death is a possibility but by sharing stories of survival—"I'm still here" and "I know others who are still here."

Breast cancer now has a high survival rate—in the United States, as high as 100 percent five-year survival for stages 0 and 1 in men and women, with an average survival of 89 percent (Fischer and Yasin, 2016; National Cancer Institute, n.d.a.). Mortality rates in the United States are decreasing, and these women need to hear that they will survive to be persuaded to feel hope. Therefore, when a member of this community (Lydia) hears from her physician that death is a possibility, she reacts emotionally, expressing her agency and denying death:

> Not a good day. . . . the plastic surgeon I saw basically outlined how I could die, step by step, for me should I choose to get reconstruction (due ot

> clots). . . . she was awful, and had me in tears. I am switching hospitals, except for my Once [oncologist].

The community members respond to this post with sympathy; none acknowledge that surgery has risks and can cause death. The members seem to focus on life (as will be addressed in the next section that addresses their expressions of gratitude) rather than on the "what if" of death. They frame their responses with *pathos*, relating to the new members' insecurities but building their *logos* by discussing the advancements in cancer treatments and decreasing mortality rates and their *ethos* by connecting with the other members, sharing their stories, and affirming the new members' concerns.

Gratitude

A diagnosis of cancer can bring a new value to and appreciation for life and to the positive things that a patient experiences every day. Faced with insecurities, patients can better cope with their diseases if they think positively (Boyles, 2007), and many patients express gratefulness and a new appreciation for life and the people around them. The need for hope is imperative and feeds the positive thinking in the community.

Community members posting in Breastcancer.org frequently express these feelings: they are thankful for a variety of subjects including life, the world, other members, and the support that they receive in the community. The most frequent expressions of gratitude are present in the "Just Diagnosed" thread, on which most members are newly diagnosed, and members share new appreciation for life:

> I do know I feel different now . . . nothing like I have ever felt before. The grass is greener the sky is bluer and I cherish every friendship with all the love I can. I am so amazed at the amount of people this disease has touched. Somehow I feel I got this to open my eyes to the REAL world (Melissa).

Helen responds, acknowledging that she too is experiencing life in a different way:

> I know what you mean—at first I felt that this was an out of the body experience. It has to be happening to someone else! Then slowly the realization came that no, it was me. You do see the world differently. And I think you listen a little closer to what people say to you. The love and encouragement from my friends has been so humbling. And you do find out who your true friends are. Some people do disappear rather quickly with the news. I take each day as it comes and enjoy my family to the max.

Both of these women share that they are learning to appreciate life and family more through their experiences with breast cancer. They are relating to each other and to other members, sharing their *pathos* but also establishing their *logos* by working through the process of appreciating life more, logically justifying their gratitude.

Several women post thanks when they ask for information, recognizing that the answer will require someone to take time to share information. For example, Stephanie shares her sister's story, asks questions, and closes her post with "Thank you for listening and for any advice you might be able to offer." Winnie also expresses appreciation in advance:

> I just read thru the forum and cried. So many emotions. I will definately be back to these pages. I know I will need the support. Does anyone know how to find local support groups? Is their a site for all support centers available? Thanks.

Many other members are also expressing "thank you" in advance (e.g., Lorraine, Linda, and Anne). These women may write "thank you" from common courtesy, which builds their *ethos* as they appreciate the community and its members; however, their statements of gratitude indicate that they appreciate each other and the support and information that they gain in the online community, an indication of their *pathos* and shared experiences.

Struggles

Women who are diagnosed will experience struggles: they are confronting a disease and pursuing complex, expensive medical care and months of cell-killing treatments with diagnostic tests and treatments from a variety of technicians and healthcare providers. The disease process of breast cancer is complex, and the members of Breastcancer.org share that complexity and their struggles with the community, seeking information, hope, empathy, and support. Other members relate: they too are going through the disease process and also are struggling. Two struggles in particular are prominent in the discourse on Breastcancer.org: financial struggles related to the cost of treatment and the unanticipated waiting that patients do during their disease process.

Financial Struggles

Costs for breast-cancer treatment can include appointments with various physicians, tests for diagnosis, surgical treatments, chemotherapy, and radiation. Costs are a great concern, and care is expensive: a 2011 study of 1444 women reported that the average costs for healthcare related to breast cancer (reporting women who underwent mastectomies and chemotherapy) ranged from $118,409 to $137,644 per patient, with costs including 29 percent for outpatient services, 26 percent for medication, 25 percent for chemotherapy drugs, and 20 percent for in-patient care during treatments (Vera-Llonch, Weycker, Glass, et al., 2011). These findings are, however, for a specific treatment plan and do not consider the diverse diagnoses, treatments, and complications that individuals diagnosed with breast cancer may experience. Other reports break down costs to specify costs for surgical treatments, chemotherapy, reconstruction, and other treatments and recovery procedures. One source estimates that surgical treatments (mastectomy and lumpectomy) can cost from $15,000 to $50,000 (CostHelper, Inc., 2017a, para. 3), and another estimates the cost for a mastectomy to be as high as $96,750 plus surgeon's fees (Mastectomy Costs, 2010). Chemotherapy can cost as little as $10,000 and as much as $100,000 with individual treatments costing $7,000 to $40,000, depending on the chemotherapy drugs and related infusion charges (CostHelper, Inc., 2017a, para. 4). On average, one chemotherapy infusion costs $18,000, and one injection of a medication to boost the patient's white blood cells can cost $15,000 (Marchione, 2012, para. 2). New chemotherapy drugs are more expensive—as much as $100,000 per year (para. 6)—as the pharmaceutical companies seek to recover research-and-development costs and because the market allows costs to rise as patients demand successful treatments.

In addition, women diagnosed with breast cancer need to decide if they want to be bald or purchase a wig and if they want to undergo reconstructive surgery or wear a prosthetic breast. A patient needs to order a wig in advance and go in to a hairdresser to choose color, cut, and style; wigs can cost as little as $30–$500 for synthetic wigs and $800–$3000 for wigs made from real human hair (Breastcancer.org, 2017). Reconstructive surgery adds additional surgical, anesthetic, and hospital expenses—as much as $150,000 for some methods (CostHelper Inc., 2017b). If a patient decides to wear an external prosthetic breast rather than undergo reconstructive surgery, she will spend between $150 and $390 for a prosthesis or $90–$550 for a form, up to $100 for other post-surgical products, and $36–$98 for a mastectomy bra (Seattle Cancer Care Alliance, 2017). A mastectomy bra is a bra that has a pocket in the side where the prosthetic or form will go; the patient can also visit a trained brasserie that can measure her for a bra from a store rack and have a tailor create a pocket for the prosthetic breast. (Often, insurance companies will cover a majority of the costs for a patient's wig and also for reconstruction or a prosthesis, charging the patient only the copay. However, if a patient is not insured or has a limited plan that does not cover these "additional" charges, she will have the additional financial burden of these appearance-related products or treatments.)

Many patients struggle to pay for medical care (Bernard, Farr, and Fang, 2011; Lauzier, Maunsell, De Koninck, et al., 2005; Markman and Luce, 2010; Szabo, 2008). A 2007 survey by the Harvard School of Public Health reports that 33 percent of cancer patients struggle to pay their medical bills, and 43 percent say they skip treatments or prescriptions because costs concern them (Gammon, 2007, para. 7). Skipping treatments and medications can create additional challenges—such as unanticipated and unnecessary side effects, less effective treatments, and decreased prescription effectiveness—and can decrease a patient's survival rate and quality of life. However, when patients are experiencing "financial toxicity" (Mulcahy, 2013), they may alleviate costs that represent what they discern are lower priorities for spending; they will delay or skip treatments that they feel they cannot afford (Harris, 2009; Markman and Luce, 2010; Szabo, 2008). As many as 10 percent of cancer patients say they cannot pay for food, shelter, and other necessities because of medical costs (Harris, 2009; Szabo, 2008). Nonprofit organizations help who they can and have seen a 30-percent increase in requests for help related to medical expenses (Szabo, 2008). The growing need from patients is increasing the burden on insurance, healthcare, and government systems (see de Kok, Dirksen, Kessels, et al., 2010; Lee, Stang, Goldberg, and Haberman, 2009).

It is no surprise that medical care costs, and it is no surprise that patients are concerned about the cost and about being able to financially survive as they seek to thrive through cancer treatments. Patients in online communities share these struggles. They may reach out to other members: to express their frustrations about the costs and to ask how to manage costs, to navigate the complex insurance system, to negotiate how to receive care, and to continue to work so they can support their families.

Community members on Breastcancer.org do disclose and discuss financial concerns and struggles. Members posting in "Progesterone Cream" discuss costs of homeopathic treatments for hormones, but they also discuss costs for physician visits and testing, asking how to make decisions related to costs. For example, Claudia asks the members to help her decide on a practitioner, based on distance, costs, and testing practices:

> I'm going to a naturopath. I have to choose between 2—one who charges $600 for the 1st visit, $175 for phone follow-ups and $225 for office follow-ups. Close to home. Uses blood for testing. And the other—charges $200 for the 1st visit, $100 follow-ups. Further from home and usees both blood and saliva. Who do I go to?

She asks other members to help her make the decision, trusting their *ethos* and expressing her *logos* by sharing her thought process and the logical approach she takes to choosing a naturopath to help her with her hormone treatment. The members who are participating in this thread of posts respond with their opinions and advise her per their experiences and preferences. Claudia does not share her final decision, but her question opens the door for other members to rhetorically participate by justifying their opinions with their own logic. Other members justify their opinions by stating that they cannot afford care: for example, Hanna shares that she cannot afford to "explore" tests and treatments that her insurance will not cover, and Carolyn acknowledges "plus its not cheap." In this way, the women also speak with *pathos* agreeing that the cost for their medical care is high and acknowledging that some members cannot afford elective (per insurance companies) tests and treatments.

Women in the midst of their treatment may not discuss the cost of medical care because they are already in the process and have other more important concerns. For example, the members posting in the "MPBC" thread focus on their diagnoses, issues with their ports, and side effects that they are experiencing; they are applying *pathos* by sharing other elements of their treatments, but they are not discussing the financial struggles. However, newly diagnosed members in the community openly discuss their concerns about finances. In "Just Diagnosed," several members openly express their concerns with continuing their work to earn an income and also with paying for medical care. For example, Lisa expresses concern that she, the family's "sole breadwinner," will not be able to work during her treatment; her post expresses her *pathos* and also her *logos*, as she explains her concern about the assumed side effects of treatment and her inability to continue to work full time and provide for her family. Janie responds with *ethos* and *logos*, sharing testimonies of other patients and explaining that Lisa can ask her physician for prescribed medications that will help her to battle side effects:

> Some people are able to still work a full time job, some have to go part time, and some have to quit until it's over. The good thing is there are so many new medications that your doctor can give you to help with many of the side affects. I think the big thing is to keep the people you work with aware of what is going on. If you are blessed and able to still work you will still need to be easy on yourself and realize your body is going through a lot right now. There are also organizations that can help with some of the medical bills. The most important thing is to make sure you take care of yourself. I know that you are probably saying to yourself that the most important thing is to keep bringing in a paycheck, but if you don't take care of you there will be no paycheck to bring in.

Lisa's concern is that she will be unable to provide for her family *and* undergo the necessary treatment for breast cancer—more about her ability to earn a living than where the money is going to go. Janie acknowledges that concern with reciprocated *pathos* and advises Lisa to take care of herself and to request financial help from some of the programs that provide if patients need help. Her *ethos* is evident by her knowledge of how to approach Lisa's concerns related to taking care of her family. Janie uses other patients' stories and her awareness of organizations that can help with a patient's financial issues (evidence) to persuade Lisa to feel hope and to find answers to Lisa's concerns.

Other members focus more on the cost of treatments rather than on their ability to earn the money to pay for those treatments—a different perspective but a similar concern. Members may voice that they are concerned because they are uninsured and thus recognize that they will carry a majority of the financial burden for their care. Two members (Ava and Brigid) are seeking Medicaid to cover the extensive costs, and Whitney is living in the United Kingdom and wondering if care will be less expensive there or in the United States. One member (Bekah) states that, because of the cost, she did not go in for a follow-up appointment:

> I have had a lump in my right breast for atleast 3 years, never going to check because of money situations, finally went to a clinic that goes by your income, and was sent right away to a clinic in Galveston [TX] where they did mammogram, ultrasound and biopsy in same day, anyways by the next week I had the results.

While this testimony may damage Bekah's *logos* within the community—because the women on this discussion board know that a lump requires immediate medical care—she builds her *pathos* with the other community members, explaining that she does not have the financial resources to pursue follow-up care. But even community members who have insurance share Bekah's concerns about the cost; they also are concerned about the control that insurance has on determining their treatments. For example, Dana, who has insurance, asks suspiciously if she can be denied care because of her coverage: "I was told I couldn't have the mamo seeds because I didn't have enough tissue. Is that true or was it my insurance?" These women have a variety of concerns, all related to the cost of care and the unknown processes related to being insured or uninsured. They address these concerns by transparently sharing their questions and concerns and by depending on the *logos* and *ethos* of other members to answer.

(The community, offering an environment of empathy, can seem to be an appropriate place to ask other patients about their financial struggles during cancer; however, the public nature of an open discussion board also creates issues of privacy and confidentiality that community members should consider. Discussing sensitive financial information can make members vulnerable—for potential fraud, for documentation of pre-existing conditions, and for other employment- and health-related conditions that typically would be considered private information. Chapter 4 will discuss issues related to self-disclosure of this information.)

Struggles with Waiting

An additional struggle with medical care is the time that is involved. Waiting is a regular part of the disease process. Some patients wait for care because they cannot afford the costs, but others wait because the healthcare system requires time for appointments, tests, results, and health communication. A patient schedules her initial appointment and waits to attend that appointment; if her caregiver suspects a diagnosis, the patient must wait as the image taken or tissue collected is tested and assessed. Diagnoses may also take multiple tests—a physician examination, a mammogram, or a CAT scan as well as biopsies. Once a patient receives a positive diagnosis, she is referred to other specialists—oncologists who provide cancer-focused treatments such as mastectomies (surgical oncologist), radiation (interventional oncologist), or chemotherapy (medical oncologist)—and she must schedule appointments with the appropriate specialists to move into treatment. After an initial meeting with the oncologist, the patient then schedules treatment (surgery, radiation, chemotherapy, or a combination in a dictated order for her customized treatment), which can include numerous appointments that span weeks or months. Even after months or years of treatment, a patient must wait while her body responds and recovers, a process that also may take a lifetime.

Waiting is a typical part of medical care; research shows that patients wait in the United States because of ethnicity (Bradley, Dahman, Shickle, and Lee, 2012); socio-economic status (Gorey, Luginaah, Holowaty, Fung, and Hamm, 2009); and demand (Bradley, Dahman, Shickle, and Lee, 2012). Patients wait in other countries because of the demand on the healthcare system—e.g., in Canada (Gorey, Luginaah, Holowaty, Fung, and Hamm, 2009) and in Nova Scotia (Saint-Jacques, Younis, Dewar, and Rayson, 2007). Patients in Nova Scotia also wait longer if they are diagnosed with earlier stages of cancer (Saint-Jacques, Younis, Dewar, and Rayson, 2007). Waiting is a difficult part of medical care for patients, and many would have decreased anxiety and increased hope as they wait if they had more information upfront about their diagnoses (Dickerson, Alquaissi, Underhill, and Lally, 2011). Patients in the United States wait because healthcare professionals have full schedules and sometimes schedule two to four weeks in advance.

The word, the discourse surrounding the term, the struggles related to waiting, and the rhetorical elements make "waiting" a part of the rhetoric of breast cancer. In online communities, members share that they struggle with the waiting—for information and for care. Waiting is particularly difficult with regard to cancer care because time allows cancer to further develop. Waiting is also difficult because of the numerous stages of treatment a patient may need to undergo during her care and because of the time required for a patient's body to recover from surgery, radiation, or chemotherapy.

Therefore, waiting for care is a challenge; patients may feel they hurry up to get a diagnosis and then wait for care and hurry up to get appointments scheduled and then wait to meet with specialists and to undergo treatment. As they wait, their disease may further develop into later stages of the disease. Therefore, they frequently express waiting as a part of their illness narrative as they share the struggles they experience.

Members in Breastcancer.org are waiting for action. For example, Mika is waiting through recovery: "Now I'm three weeks out since my finale tx and patiently (yea right) waiting for my hair to grow back." (For many patients, when their hair begins to grow, they know that their bodies are beginning to recover from chemotherapy. Thus, hair is a sign of hope and of coming closure.) Other members struggle with waiting to learn more about their diagnoses and treatments and waiting to have their cancer removed. For example, Lydia learns her diagnosis but, because of the holidays, she must wait to begin treatment:

> Since I was diagnosed in December, then had to wait 2 weeks to get in to the big university hospital here, I ran into a problem with Christmas and surgeons being off for 2 weeks. . . . it was horrible to have to wait, knowing that lump was there all through the holidays.

Similarly, Natalie is frustrated because she must wait to learn what her healthcare provider will suggest as treatment:

> The Dr. also said she didn't know if they would do the surgery first or start the chemo. . . . So now I have to wait until Wednesday to get more info on my next chapter, which sucks. . . I wanted it like now!

Responding to Natalie, Michele responds with empathy:

> I'm so sorry you have to go through this stressful period waiting for information about your bc. . . . I had to wait 3 days while they figured out the type [of my breast cancer]. Those were the longest 3 days of my life. Then there was another 4 days waiting for the appointment. . . . I'll be thinking about you and wishing you peace during this difficult waiting period.

Members express *pathos* as they empathetically share their own experiences with waiting for diagnostic information and then with treatment to begin. These women share the struggle and express, "I will be thinking of you." The members' discourse does not address *logos*; the women do not justify the wait. They all share frustration about waiting and do not see the logic of waiting for data or treatment because healthcare providers cannot see them immediately.

Some women choose to wait: because of financial duress or because they need to feel some control and thus fit their scheduled appointments into their schedules. One member, Lora, chooses to wait, posting, "I may wait for radiation I was also told that I probably have it on the other side as well." Waiting may help members feel like they have some agency; they may need the control in the process to make decisions. Others may need to wait, finding that surging ahead can create more stress. For example, Whitney determines to wait to research her diagnoses—"I know reading stuff online has been frightening to me. Maybe I should wait to research after I know more."—to which Adrian replies, with *logos*, "Please limit your research to sites like this or other valid ones, and yes, wait till you have some good info about YOUR pathology before overloading yourself with information that will certainly keep you up nights!" Patients who wait to research potential diagnoses and treatments may save themselves the stress of wondering "what if" before they know the details about their own diagnoses and thus may be more easily persuaded to embrace hope.

Other community members wait because they need specialized medications that are not readily available. Most chemotherapy drugs as well as those for surgical procedures and side effectives are readily available, but some specialized drugs must be specially ordered—perhaps they are not readily prescribed or are new drugs that are just coming out of the research-and-development process—and patients then need to wait until their providers can access the necessary medications. For example, Jeri shares a situation related to her waiting for a medication:

> I am concerned about the delay and my surgeon's office said they are waiting to hear from the hospital as to when the next shipment [of the drug needed] will be received.

Jeri posts the only message that expresses indefinite waiting; most members wait but have an idea of how long they will be waiting. Therefore, most of the references to waiting include an end, such as when the patient will have an appointment, start treatment, or have surgery. This particular post expresses a member's concern about waiting for her treatment—to start her medication. Waiting for medication can be a part of the disease process for transplant surgery or for medications related to flu or viruses when the medications are finishing the development stage; however, waiting for medication is not typical for patients seeking treatment for breast cancer. Jeri does not ask questions about her wait; she expresses her concern without providing details, but *logos* illuminates that she is concerned because she needs to start treatment and she does not know how long she will need to wait.

Waiting can cause frustration, concern, and duress, and community members may share their feelings in their discourse, anticipating that other community members will understand and express *pathos*. For example, Ava posts, "The waiting is really getting to me. I want to begin fighting this alien inside me," and Roma expresses similar frustration:

> I think the not knowing and the waiting is what drives me crazy, I hate the weekend as can't find out anything. . . . I have never been scared so far, the frustration has been the waiting in between.

Mary states,

> [This is] the hardest part of the journey—the waiting. Once you know what you are dealing with and have a treatment plan in place it does get easier.

These women know their diagnoses but are in the process of waiting for their providers' or hospital schedules. They share their responses to waiting in the online community and are able, as a part of the rhetoric of breast cancer, to relate to others who are waiting. They understand the repercussions of waiting for treatment and may be concerned that their cancer will progress during the wait; they also share the feeling of anxiety to remove or destroy the cancer. Within the community, they must depend on shared stories and evidence that a few weeks will not change their diagnoses or the outcome of their treatments.

Disease Names

The rhetoric of a disease is incomplete without a discussion about how the patients refer to their disease. Patients have freedom in naming their disease, whereas their healthcare providers do not. Providers use terms that they have learned through their education and professional experiences; they seek to use medical terminology to reference a disease, seeking to be accurate and to eliminate ambiguity that might create chaos in their communication with other providers. They also use accurate and established terms when discussing disease with patients to ensure that they communicate per standard terms, eliminating misunderstandings and thus being liable for inaccurate or unclear communication. Patients, however, have the freedom to use terms that relate to their personal experiences; they do not need to worry about anyone else knowing the exact diagnoses they have received. They may use medical jargon to reference the processes they are experiencing, but they may also apply rhetorical devices to more accurately label their disease and to express their experiences with others who are experiencing the same. They may apply experience, metaphor, or humor to determine the names for their disease. The names that they assign to their disease or to their tumors may be a valuable part of their disease narrative, including a personalized experience or feeling that they share with the other members in building their place in the community. Research shows that patients use personal terms for breast cancer—terms like "monster" or "beast" (Radin, 2006, p. 594). In this way, patients can frame their discourse with personal references and integrate into the rhetoric of breast cancer terms that include their experiences. But in the community on Breastcancer.org, the members also use other terms.

Members in Breastcancer.org use established terms for their disease—such as "breast cancer," "cancer," "BC," or other standard phrases and words—as they seek to communicate clearly with globally understood and accepted terms. They also seek to learn what is understood; for example, Michele clarifies what she is referencing in a previous post: "BTW, I've started using MPBC rather than MBC to distinguish it [metaplastic breast cancer] from metastatic breast cancer. You think that's OK, or are there certain acronyms we are supposed to use." Michele is aware that some medical terms are more readily accepted, and she wants to ensure that she was communicating effectively. She asks the members of the community if her abbreviation is okay and asks if she should use some other term. She submits herself to the community to learn the term and ensure that she is clearly communicating her disease type. In response to Michele's question, Katie responds similarly:

> Might mbc be thought of by some as metastisis bc, or is that how it's defined in my mind only? I lean toward keeping the mpbc acronym, but, whatever is most suitable and helpful to others that may come behind us is what's important . . . . you are the veterans,here. . . . what do you think is best?

These women are asking about disease-specific terms to ensure that they are speaking the rhetoric of breast cancer and communicating effectively with other members. But they also affirm the *ethos* of the other members, stating that others are "veterans" and they would know more. Also, both Michele and Katie *ask* about the term for their type of cancer; they explain their logic behind the names they are using, but they then petition the more experienced members of the community by asking what is best and what is correct. This further affirms that members come to this community because they believe that the members know and they feel welcome to ask questions.

On Breastcancer.org, newly diagnosed women posting in "Just Diagnosed" refer to their diagnoses as "breast cancer" or with terms that are established and used by medical professionals who have diagnosed the disease. However, members who have been diagnosed and are undergoing treatment may label their disease and its role in their lives: the "journey," the "beast," or the magically appearing mass. They establish their own terms for cancer and for elements related to cancer—to integrate humor into their discourse, to express their feelings about their diagnoses, and to share their experiences. For example, Carolyn (posting in the thread called "Progesterone Cream") writes, "lesion, mass, tumor, don't all those words just suck! I like 'blip' a little blip doesn't sound so scary!" As she states, she is seeking to decrease the fear she feels when she hears medical jargon related to her tumor, and she is using humor and a minimizing word—"blip"—to diminish the thread of the words that the medical professionals use. Other community members understand and apply metaphors: Katie refers to breast cancer as "this 'c' thing," "beast," and the "dark cloud." She minimizes the seriousness of the situation by not calling it by name and even using metaphors to parallel what the disease is doing in her life. Natalie also calls it the "beast." And Natalie takes her metaphor further by referring to her tumor as "Houdini," in reference to the illusionist who escaped locks and sealed boxes ("Harry Houdini Dies," 2010) and thus using the metaphor for her mass, which she found nine months after her annual mammogram. She explains, "I just can't figure out when [Houdini] . . . showed up." Natalie uses humor in sharing this story, minimizing how a tumor can show up between mammogram appointments and instead making light by naming her tumor. In this way, she connects with those who are seeking to gain hope (and those who are persuading other members to feel hope).

The online members of Breastcancer.org also use the term *NED* in their discourse. This term is explained by a member, Virginia, who has posted 3,291 times in the community. Virginia writes,

> You will read about people dancing with NED here a lot. Although I'm sure that there's a fella named NED out there somewhere who is quite a dancer, the NED we're talking about is NO EVIDENCE OF DISEASE. I haven't had the opportunity to dance with him yet, but only because he's been very busy dancing with others. I'm sure my turn will come eventually!

NED is a term that members use throughout the online community on Breastcancer.org. The more experienced members are looking forward to "dancing with NED," but the newer members relate to the desire for NED and see NED as a shared landmark for all members. Their hope is to reach NED, and the more members who share that they "dance with NED," the more evidence that the women will, at some point in the future, be told that their PET scans show no evidence of breast cancer. The rhetorical value of NED—the logical justification of NED as a realistic future, the shared desire for a dance with NED, and the members' desire that their community friends will also dance with NED—is great in the rhetoric of breast cancer.

The Rhetoric of Breast Cancer in Online Discourse

Women diagnosed with breast cancer integrate its rhetoric into their communication, and if they are members of an online community like Breastcancer.org, they may learn the language and communication methods around their disease from others who are experiencing the same disease process. This rhetoric can include the expression of feelings, discourse about struggles, and personalized terms for the disease.

The rhetoric of breast cancer also includes patient discourse related to the patients' experiences and opinions of the U.S. medical system, particularly their treatments, their healthcare providers, and sometimes even pharmaceutical companies, insurance companies, and medical researchers (addressed in chapter 3).

NOTES

1. The two Web sites have been moved to www.Breastcancer.org/symptoms/understand_bc/fears/managing.jsp and www.Breastcancer.org/symptoms/diagnosis/index.jsp, respectively.
2. I have changed dates in posts to 00/00/0000 (or a format similar to the original content) to protect the creators of the posts, as diagnoses, treatment, reconstruction, and appointment dates may be identifying information.

Chapter Three

Patients, Medical Care, and Rhetoric

Healthcare providers speak about providing medical care for patients; they interact with each other differently than they do with their patients (Barton, 2004). They use the voice of medicine, through medical rhetoric, and include medical terminology, objective analysis of measurable and reported evidence, and a categorization of symptoms and equation of diagnoses as they relate to basic sciences and a "biomedical model" (Charles, Gafni, and Whelan, 2000, p. 1). They interact as they are taught in their medical training, speaking as professionals who sometimes must separate themselves from their work. For providers, medicine is work.

Healthcare providers and patients interact with each other with a unique and different rhetoric, centering on the classification of symptoms but framing their discourse with a focus on the patient's well-being and the healthcare provider's experience and responsibility to provide knowledge and care. Their interaction is typically adapted per the patient's level of understanding and of participation; the healthcare provider will shift the rhetoric to meet the patient's needs and expectations because the patient has less flexibility. The patient's understanding is a variable within the interaction that should affect both parties.

And patients communicate with other patients using a different rhetoric—with an empathetic and understanding tone (*pathos*); a communal voice with information, credibility, and resources from their research (*ethos*); and a logical medical focus (*logos*) that allows them to express their agency and together seek to be an active part of the medical community. Patients communicate in face-to face support meetings but also via media in virtual spaces (such as the discussion board on Breastcancer.org, although many other online communities do and will exist). Patients who are active members of the online communities share their narratives, perhaps not as scholars consider traditional narratives but as are relevant in the digital age. The discourse of patients in these online spaces adds dimension to the rhetoric of their diseases and gives us another perspective—a dialect, if you will—of the rhetoric of health and medicine. The dialect on Breastcancer.org is the rhetoric of breast cancer.

Rhetorical scholars and researchers study the back-stage (with other physicians) discourse of physicians (Barton, 2004) and the front-stage discourse of physicians with patients (e.g., see Alkureishi, Lee, Lyons, et al., 2016; Bertakis, 2009; Cousin, Mast, Roter, and Hall, 2012; Gáspárik, Ábrám, Geana, et al., 2014; Ishikawa, Hashimoto, and Kuichi, 2013; Klitzman, 2006; Paternotte, van Dulmen, van der Lee, Scherpbier, Schelle, 2015; Smith, Guyton, Pariser, et al., 2016; Talen, Grampp, Tucker, and Schultz, 2008; Tsai, Lu, and Frankel, 2013). However, patient-to-patient discourse is frequently overlooked, even though communication between patients is an important part of medical discourse. What, why, and how patients are discussing and sharing provides the medical community with an additional, and valuable, element of patient "back-stage" discourse (to use Barton's [2004] term). If researchers and scholars are going to analyze patient-to-patient discourse, they must investigate how members of online communities converse, not only about their diagnoses and their diseases but also about medicine, health, their healthcare providers, and other processes and elements that directly relate to the medical community. "Besides [seeking] diagnostic and treatment [information], they [patients] seek details about scientific discovery, alternative approaches, continuing care, rehabilitation, and even the politics of breast cancer" (Radin, 2006, pp. 594–95). Therefore, analysis of these communities helps communicators to consider how patients use online communities to construct their experiences with diseases and helps healthcare providers better know what patients want, need, and experience during their disease processes. As stated in the introduction of this book, patient discourse has a place in the rhetorics of health and medicine (e.g., references in Arduser, 2017; Keränen, 2010; Meloncon and Frost, 2015; Segal, 2005; and Seigel, 2013) and in the discourse within the medical community (e.g., Mol's [2002] theory of inclusion). Segal (2005) encourages rhetorical scholars and researchers to consider patient discourse, "not a particular text but rather a discourse as a whole" (p. 5). Therefore, researchers can look at the sentences and topics of patients' expressions (such as the posts that I am analyzing) but also consider their motives and the context of the discourse within the community and the conversation where the discourse exists.

Historically, when individuals became ill or experienced symptoms that concerned them, they consulted with a physician to determine their diagnoses. They visited a physician's office (or the physician visited the patients at home when physicians made house calls) to ask and answer questions, and the patients, trusting the physician, complied with the healthcare provider's instructions and treatment plans. Medicine at that time centered around the physician's texts in practice—notes, books, reports, interviews, and records (Derkatch and Segal, 2005). In consulting with a physician, a patient provided a narrative of illness—a report of symptoms and the story of how the disease affects life—and the physician completed the narrative by identifying the patient's disease and determining the best course of action to deal with that diagnosis. However, medicine is changing. As medicine becomes less paternalistic and more patient-centered, and as patient–physician communication is emphasized as an important skill that practitioners need, patients are empowered to participate in the decision-making process, to determine how they deal with their diagnoses, and to speak up about the medical care that they receive. These changes allow patients to participate in their medical care and to be part of the multiple realities of illness, as Mol (2002) investigates in her ethnographic study of atherosclerosis and patients. Whereas healthcare providers focus on the disease, the diagnosis, and solving the problems related to the dysfunction in the patient's body, the patient focuses on disease and diagnosis as well as on the elements of disease that affects life, giving the consideration of disease a new, wider, and more personalized perspective of illness. This expanded perspective allows a patient to be considered as a person, not only as a vessel that carries the bacteria, virus, or dysfunctional cells or as the face of disease. A patient is then empowered to express agency: to ask questions, make decisions, and take control of the disease process. She is encouraged to develop and express agency as she shares her illness narrative.

Americans are increasingly using the World Wide Web for health and medical information (Bunde, Suis, Martin, and Barnett, 2006; Cline and Haynes, 2001; Finfgeld, 2000; Whitten, Smith, Munday, and LaPlante, 2008). Technology has expanded how individuals learn about their symptoms and diagnoses. But technology has also expanded how patients construct their illness narratives and express agency. Patients may complete surveys as they walk out of their physicians' offices or provide patient feedback in review pages (e.g., Healthgrades, ZocDoc, RateMDs, and Vitals). They can also share their experiences in online communities: in addition to discoursing with other patients and sharing their experiences, they can express satisfaction and dissatisfaction; share concerns; ask questions; and encourage others to express their agency and manage their healthcare by choosing providers, dealing with insurance, and considering how healthcare policy and the U.S. healthcare system affect their care and their illness narratives. They participate in the rhetoric of that community, discussing shared experiences and concerns, influencing how others perceive their identities by building credibility, and analyzing circumstances together to make logical decisions about their healthcare. In these spaces, patients also encourage each other to control their experiences: to ask questions if they want to know something or if something does not make sense, to get second and even third opinions on their diagnoses and treatment plans, to change healthcare providers if they have questions or are dissatisfied, and to feel free to criticize care that they feel is less than it should be.

These online communities are a rich source of patients' research and resources and of their experiential data. "This collective intelligence should be evaluated, not simply dismissed as amateur, unreliable, and possibly even malicious. The medical information monopoly is dead, and how constructively medical professionals accept this will help to determine how widely society will benefit from the new order" (Radin, 2006, p. 600). This new order allows patients to ask questions and share information about their treatments, to discourse about insurance, to question pharmaceutical companies and the research and development process of drugs, and to reflect on their healthcare providers: their primary care providers, surgeons, oncologists, radiologists, nurses, technicians, and other professionals who are responsible for their treatments. For women who are members of Breastcancer.org, the online community provides a "safe" place where they can focus on life that surrounds that disease—how to survive, thrive, and recover.

This chapter focuses on the patient-to-patient discourse on the discussion board of Breastcancer.org that relates to the community members' experience within the medical community and to the rhetoric of breast cancer.

PATIENT DISCOURSE ABOUT TREATMENTS

Patient communities may perpetuate inaccurate information (as discussed in chapter 2), but community discourse more frequently contains accurate information and patient discourse that focuses on patients' experiences and research. Thus, these communities are valuable resources for patients who are seeking information about treatments from a patient perspective. Members in these online communities are researching their own diagnoses and treatments—for their own benefit as well as the benefit of the other members of community. Whereas they share their own disease narratives and the information that their healthcare providers share with them, they also share empirical information to support their healthcare decisions. As a result, patients in these online communities bring together research and methods from different fields and different philosophies—such as osteopathic, naturopathic, medicinal, holistic, and traditional (alternative)—to share different studies with different hypotheses and different approaches to treatment. In Breastcancer.org, the members follow this theory and bring together information and research from different treatment philosophies, potentially creating some conflict in the information that the members of the community share but seeking as individuals to build their *ethos* and *logos* within the community by sharing experiences and resources that support their narratives and their treatment decisions. The comments on care that they share may not align because the approaches to treatment are so different.

The thread called "Progesterone Cream" illustrates this conflict between different approaches to and the patients' inquiries about effective treatment. Started by a member asking, "Is anyone using progesterone cream to help balance hormone levels?" (Karen), this thread contains 469 posts published by women who share their questions, experiences, and resources about homeopathic treatments for hormone imbalance with side references to treatments from medical physicians who are practicing per evidence and findings in research within the basic sciences. These women are investigating their treatments and potential treatments, seeking to know about their bodies and their options. In sharing information, women posting in "Progesterone Cream" share resources and discuss the treatments they are receiving to together create a full spectrum of opportunities that the members can consider for treatment. For example, Kristi explains to a member the differences between a prescription and a compound that other members are discussing:

> your doc is prescribing synthetic progesterone (Provera, also known as MPA methroxyprogesterone acetate). That causes the side effects and even can suppress your body's own natural progesterone. It is horrible. There is no way natural progesterone causes clots. Even estrogen doesn't cause clots as long as it isn't given orally. That has been researched in France where a large part of the population uses progesterone and estrogen in gel form.

Kristi then charges the other members to consider international research and to read: "We all have to read more than our doctors." And six posts later, she writes, "I've done bioidenticals for years. My PCP [primary care practitioner] knows I won't do anything that I haven't researched thoroughly." And just a few posts later, she answers Julia's question, "what is an observational study?" with a post:

> An observational study is a study where they look [at] a group of people who did one thing and compare that group with another group that did something else. They observe what happened after the fact. . . . In the "randomized, double blind, placebo-controlled" studies (which are considered more prestgious) you get a pill and neither you nor your doctor know if you're getting the drug or the placebo. Then at the end the study is "unblended" and you find out if you were getting the placebo or not.

Kristi is one of the members who researches carefully to ensure the accuracy of her information—for herself and also for the benefit of the other members in this online community. She establishes her credibility (her *ethos*) with the members who are discoursing in this thread by using the compound name of

Provera, by referring to international research on progesterone, by sharing that she has used bioidenticals "for years," by establishing that her primary care provider is aware of what she is doing, and by explaining how research is conducted (using medical terms like "observational study" and "randomized, double blind, placebo-controlled" studies). Kristi does not identify herself as a member of the medical profession; however, she does share information that illustrates her credibility as an informed patient. She also illustrates her *logos* by identifying that she understands the logical process of clotting and the standards of an observational study. However, in expressing her knowledge, she does not eliminate *pathos*: she maintains her place as one of the women who is learning how to use progesterone cream by using "we" and by challenging the other members to read more than their physicians. In her tone, language, and inclusive pronoun, she establishes that she is one of the patients within this community; she is "one of them" on Breastcancer.org.

Another member, Ruth, shares information about her treatment for hormone imbalance:

> To get this far it has taken me two months of discussion with my Gyno, Onc, saliva test, Pharmacist etc. My saliva test result showed Prog=.5, Test=16 and Cortisol=2.1 (morning) and I will need to monitor my Cortisol in the future as it is extremely low at which is the high point of the day.

Ruth also builds her *logos*, *ethos*, and *pathos* through the information she shares and the tone with which she shares that data. She shares the logical process that she will need to follow to measure her hormones in her saliva. Ruth builds her *ethos*—her credibility as an informed patient and informative member of the community—by sharing her test scores with labels and what she needs to do. She knows what she is doing, and she has conversed with her healthcare providers to learn about the saliva test to monitor her cortisol levels. She builds her *pathos* by maintaining her status as a patient and addressing her discussions with her healthcare providers (her gynecologist, her oncologist, and her pharmacist) as the other community members are doing. In this, the other patients know that she is a patient who is also seeking to get answers to her questions. Ruth shares her tests and chosen treatment with great detail—to justify her decision and also to inform other women about how she has made choices and been involved in her treatment (*logos*).

In the "MPBC" thread, the members share about their treatments for metaplastic breast cancer, although they do not support their information with personally accessed resources but with experience only. The six women share the same diagnosis and thus may not need to support their information as much as members discoursing in larger groups. However, these women do discourse in this thread about their medicinal treatments, particularly the drugs they are receiving and their experiences with tests and ports. In this way, the women connect and individually build their *ethos* and *pathos*: by specifying their treatments and sharing experiences that parallel what the other women posting in the thread have experienced. They share specific information about their chemotherapy drugs (42 general and 15 specific references), diagnostic tests (41 general and 15 specific references), members' ports (26 references), and test results (24 references). They also discuss their surgical treatments with technical medical terms—e.g.,

- bilateral mastectomy (Lydia),
- lumpectomy (Natalie),
- mammogram (Natalie) and mammo (Michele),
- intubated (Michele),
- ultrasounds (Natalie),
- needle biopsy (Katie), and
- partial mastectomy (Katharine).

In this way, they share their treatment regimens with credibility, connecting them together as a community, even though they have not all undergone identical treatments.

In discussing their treatments, the members use general terms—like "surgery" and "scans" and references to needles being inserted into ports or veins (discussed below). They also refer to their chemical treatments as "chemo" (rather than "chemotherapy") except in one post, in which Katie calls chemotherapy the "IV poison" (and then apologizes for her humor—integrating *pathos* into her narrative by ensuring that she does not offend anyone with her joke). These women share specific information about their treatments in their discussions. For example, two of the six members posting in this thread know and reference their chemotherapy drugs by market name and share their regimens:

- Lydia is taking "TC" (nonanthracycline adjuvant docetaxel/cyclophosphamide; Nierengarten, 2005); "AC/Taxol" (adriamycin and cyclophosphamide followed by administration of Taxol (Cancernet–uk, n.d.); tamoxifen; and "AI" (aromatase inhibitors; Breastcancer.org, 2011); and
- Katherine is taking "FEC" (a combination of fluorouracil, epirubicin, and cyclophosphamide; Cancerhelp UK, 2010); Taxotere (docetaxel injection; PubMed Health, n.d.); and Zometa (zoledronic acid injection; PubMed Health, 2011).

These women discuss their medications per market names but without explaining what the drugs do; the other members respond as if they know about these medications and do not need explanation, a sign that the members are relating to and understanding each other.

In this thread of posts, the members encourage each other to save copies of medical records so they can document their treatments in detail, explaining how they are obtaining detailed treatment information and showing that they consider those records to gather information about their own treatments. In this way, they encourage each other to build their *ethos* by arming themselves with their own medical information.

Perhaps the most telling care-related discourse in this online community is twenty-six instances in the thirty-one posts in the "MPBC" thread when members specifically address treatments related to their ports. A port is an insertion site that is surgically created for the duration of a treatment; it is a "port" of entry—an implant that allows for drug infusion or blood extraction, eliminating the need of perpetual needle sticks, insertion for a larger needle, and thus safety (less infection) and comfort (less pain) for the patient. The women communing through posts in the "MPBC" thread discuss their experiences related to their ports: placement, insertion of needles, and complications. Three of the women post about the pain they experience during needle insertion, and they ask how the other members deal with the pain, never referencing their healthcare providers. They share their pain, expanding the *pathos* in the thread because the women relate to the pain of needle insertion into ports and directly into their tissues and muscles. The women also establish *logos* in their discussion by logically addressing the process of dealing with the pain related to needle insertion in ports.

First, Katie posts that she has undergone placement of her port, and Mika responds:

> don't they numb the area before they insert the needle? If they don't you should ask them to.I'm so glad I did the port thing, as the chemo has the potential to damage your veins. I will have mine [port] for a while as I'm seeing my onc [oncologist] every 6 weeks for blood work and I have to talk to him about what comes next. I was looking at my adinum lab work for E R,PR and HER, and found that my ER is now 1–5% positive where on the original they were all neg[negative]. [1]

Mika shares her experiences with medical terms that are specific to her treatment and her experience, and she logically addresses the process of her thinking about this post. In particular, she uses jargon such as "ER" to refer to "estrogen receptor" (a term that would mean "emergency room" in other medical rhetorics but that refers to breast-cancer-specific terms in this subset of the medical community), "PR" for "progesterone receptor," and "HER" for "human epidermal growth factor receptor" (a gene that can add to breast-cancer development). Using these terms Mika shows that she knows about her disease and the terms within the context of breast cancer. Mika then starts with a question to Katie about her pain, and she recommends a way to deal with the pain, giving Katie permission to ask for a local anesthetic the next time she undergoes needle insertion into her port. Thus, she affirms Katie's pain, answers her question, and gives additional information in a credible and knowing manner.

The women posting in the "MPBC" thread are in the midst of their treatments; in contrast, the newly diagnosed members posting in "Just Diagnosed" thread are those who have recently been diagnosed with breast cancer and experienced community members who respond to the questions from the new community members. In the 176 posts in the "Just Diagnosed" thread, members reference a variety of tests and treatments:

- general tests (82 times);
- pathology reports (31 times);
- treatments (25 general references with
    - 125 references to surgical treatments,
    - 49 to chemotherapy,
    - 47 to radiation, and
    - 11 to hormone therapy); and
- reconstruction (20 times).

These women are learning about their new diagnoses and sharing information about their diagnostic tests and early conversations with their providers, most likely so the patients feel control over their information and thus their circumstances. They may also seek to connect with others who share their diagnoses because the newly diagnosed members recognize the *ethos* of the community and are seeking information, assurance, and hope from those who have "gone before them"—an important element in the breast-cancer community and in the rhetoric of breast cancer.

These women also reference their cancer diagnoses (137 instances) with detailed notes, including

- "'poorly differentiated infiltrating ductal carcinoma' Histolgic grade 3. Metastatic to lymph node" (Tisha);
- "stage 3A,T3 cancer of the left breast" (Emily);
- "2 atypical ductal hyperplasia tumors . . . 3.1x2.6 cent size . . . 'high-grade infiltrating ductal carcinoma'" (Konstanze);
- "grade 2 infiltrating duct cancer i have DCIS [Ductal Carcinoma *In Situ*] that is solid, cribroform and comedo—mass size 1.9x1.2x1cm" (Holly); and
- "invasive lobular carcinoma" (Cyndi).

They do not state "I have breast cancer" but instead provide specific information about the diseases they are fighting. In this way, they share that they know what type of breast cancer they are confronting (an action that builds their credibility within the community) and also a way to connect with others who have shared the same diagnoses and who can empathize.

In response to the growing ethos of the newly diagnosed members, the experienced members share advice, practicing their already established *ethos* as members of Breastcancer.org and expressing *pathos* for the newly diagnosed members to assure the new members that they understand and to give the new members hope. For example, Bridgett posts, "Understanding your treatment will help you deal with the fear of the unknown" and Cathy adds her own advice, also seeking to persuade the new members to feel hope: "you will find many of us on that threat that have finished treatment and feel great, positive and very optimistic." Most of the members post about their specific treatments: lumpectomies (e.g., Gail, Melissa, and Stephanie) and mastectomies (e.g., Becky, Virginia, and Holly). And some members are even more detailed in establishing their credibility with more detail about their experience:

- Emily—"I had a modified radical mastectomy with sentinel node biopsy."
- Merlene—"I had a mammotome biopsy—with I think is the same as a core biopsy and they placed a titanium chip at the biopsy site to make it easier to find the place to do the lumpectomy if needed. This way they know exactly where the samples came from."
- Debbie—"I had my lumpectomy . . . with sentinel node biopsy."

By sharing details, these women seek to belong by sharing their "qualifications": they too have undergone the initial surgical treatments for breast cancer and thus are a part of the greater community of breast-cancer patients, but they are also seeking to qualify to be a part of the community on Breastcancer.org by using medical terms that the other patients will understand. Not all of these members ask questions; some of them are introducing themselves with the credibility established by their scars.

Many of the members will also undergo chemotherapy treatment, using "chemo" and "chemotherapy" to refer to this treatment, and some will also undergo radiation, an experience they also share:

- Merlene—"The radiation is placed into the area where the calcifications were removed through a balloon that is placed into the breast during the surgery rather than 30 sessions of external radiation. This treatment is new and no longer experimental. It has been used for over 10 years."

- Nina—"I though that aromatase therapy was given after tamoxifen. I was hoping to just have radiation. The side effects are not as bad as tamoxifen, but still (osteoporosis, bone pain, elevated cholesterol)."

Other references to radiation and other therapies are general but include details like the length of treatment or the type of cancer with which they have been diagnosed. In all of this discourse, the experienced members are discoursing within the *ethos* that they have established and the *pathos* that they seek to develop between community members, and the newly diagnosed members are introducing themselves, using specific terminology and the same tone as the other members are using to introduce themselves. (Some of the newly diagnosed members express their initial feelings of fear, as presented in chapter 2. But some newly diagnosed members introduce themselves with their diagnoses, guarding their emotions and seeking to build relationships within the community but moving forward slowly to establish trust and to test the credibility of other members.)

In this way, the patients openly discourse about their treatments. They treat the procedures they have undergone as qualifications for them to be accepted and included. The community does share a purpose (as noted in chapter 1), and as individuals introduce themselves and share their diagnoses and treatments, the breast-cancer patients are justified as members of the community. They are welcomed by already established members, and they accept membership (without choice about their diagnoses but by choice in their action in Breastcancer.org) with posts between members that say, "I'm so glad you found us" and "I'm glad I found y'all" (Virginia, Melissa, Konstanze, and Hayley). Members then use terms like "sisters" (Katie and Lydia) or "club" to explain the feeling of the group. As Margaret explains, "I have heard and have used these words . . . 'This is a club that nobody would choose to join.' It is a club of fabulous women and some men. I feel a special connection to every woman that has ever experienced breast cancer." Other members refer to community of breast-cancer patients as "the club none of us wanted to join" (Janie) and the "club nobody wants to join" (Stacy), and Charity explains membership best: "To all, your stories are heroic to say the very least. I didn't choose this club, but I'm proud to be associated with all of you." The connection—the *pathos*—is evident in language that is inclusive for a community of those who share a diagnosis. These women include their relationships with other breast-cancer patients as a part of their illness narratives, no matter what specific breast-cancer diagnosis and disease-specific treatments the members experience.

PATIENT DISCOURSE ABOUT INSURANCE

Women in the community of Breastcancer.org do not focus most of their discourse on the U.S. insurance system. However, they do address insurance companies as one category of agencies that they must consider as they pursue care. Their discourse is both negative and positive, depending on the members' experiences.

Three members posting in the "Progesterone Cream" thread share criticism of insurance. Marty states that she is experimenting with iodine and myomine as part of her hormone-imbalance treatments, and after she tests her hormone levels, she will attend a meeting to "campaign" for Blue Cross, a large U.S. insurance company, to cover tests and preventative treatments; however, she anticipates that the insurance company will not respond positively to her campaign, saying, "I can dream can't I?" She shares that she is experimenting, not within a research study but testing on herself. Thus, she seeks to *create* evidence that will increase her credibility outside the community. She will then take that evidence to her insurance company to advocate for coverage for patients who are seeking to use these substances as treatment for hormone imbalance. She is not doing this only for herself but is petitioning for the insurance company to cover *all* of its patients who might benefit from this treatment. Marty's discourse in this community tells a deeper story: her critical thinking tells her (*logos*) that Blue Cross will not listen or respond to her petition unless she establishes some credibility (*ethos*), but her *pathos*—her compassion and care for other patients who are experiencing what she is experiencing and who need these treatments—drives her to consider petitioning the insurance company to persuade the company to cover the treatments, even if she knows that the battle for coverage might be lost.

Hanna shares in her post that she cannot try progesterone cream because her insurance company will not cover the expense for the treatment. She is then participating in the thread of posts to see what other members are sharing. Hanna is seeking affordable (or covered) treatments that she can try to improve the quality of her life, and through her discourse, she insinuates a need (supported by her *pathos* and *ethos*) for insurance-covered treatment and a respect for the community on Breastcancer.org as she seeks suggestions and hope. As Hanna does, Claudia shares that her insurance company will not cover her care through a naturopathic doctor because the company does not include naturopaths in the list of covered providers. Both women share the limits of their insurance, but neither takes the rhetoric beyond the statements of their coverage limitations; they do not petition for ideas or propose advocacy, as Marty does. However, their presence within the community illustrates that they are participating in the rhetoric: they acknowledge that the community members are credible, sharing information that might benefit them, and they then participate to belong, to gather information, to empathize (and receive empathy), or to experience a combination of these purposes.

Advocacy is a potential action for members who are participating in the community and who engage in the rhetoric of breast cancer. Other communities do have members who advocate; "In the course of mutual support, it is only natural that some will identify targets for social action, from poor hospital procedures to environmental poisons. Thus, a community can, in its unstudied way, deal with issues of social policy" (Radin, 2006, p. 592). Breastcancer.org may include more community members who are advocating and dealing with policy issues, as Marty expresses.

Community members, particularly members who are posting in the thread titled "Progesterone Cream," also share positive comments about their insurance companies. Two members, Ruth and Gwenn, post positive reports about what their insurance covers. Ruth states that her prescriptions for hormone tests, progesterone, and testosterone are covered by her insurance company, and she only pays her copay. By sharing, she is expressing satisfaction that she can access treatment that her insurance approves and covers; she is then freed of some of the financial struggles related to medical care (and discussed in chapter 2).

Gwenn also has a positive experience with her insurance:

> Tah Dah!!!! Not only did I find a REAL doctor that my insurance will pay for me to see. She is pro-homeopathic and does BHRT [bioidentical hormone replacement therapy]. She will send Rx's [prescriptions] to a compounding pharmacy. . . . She will test all of my hormones & since I have period [menstrual cycle] issues she said some meds may be covered by my insurance! . . . I know my insurance won't pay for all the Rx's . . . but she is a doctor & they will pay for me to have a PCP [primary care provider].

Gwenn visits her physician for the first time and returns to the community to report, "AND my insurance paid for her because she is a REAL doctor!" Gwenn does not explain what she means when she describes her physician as a "REAL doctor," but her references to a physician who considers homeopathic treatments, who prescribes prescriptions covered by insurance, and who is covered by insurance (and thus approved) indicate qualifications for a physician to be "REAL." (Gwenn does not mention her physician's education, post-graduate training, licensure, or years in the practice when she defines her physician as being "REAL.") Gwenn then goes further than Ruth, who expressed satisfaction that her insurance covers her tests. Gwenn begins her post with "Tah Dah!!!," a reference to magic and the unexpected, inferring that she is surprised.

PATIENT DISCOURSE ABOUT PHARMACEUTICAL COMPANIES

Perhaps the most common medicinal treatment for breast cancer is chemotherapy, which is the infusion of chemical compounds that interrupt the multiplication of cells. Thus, cancer cells are stopped, but fast-growing cells (such as those in fingernails, hair, and tissue inside the mouth) are also interrupted. Because chemotherapy is a standard treatment for many types of breast cancer, patients who are diagnosed with a form of the disease anticipate that they will undergo chemotherapy.

Chemotherapy drugs are researched and developed by pharmaceutical companies around the world. The drugs are expensive because the research-and-development process is costly; the companies pay for costs—including supplies, personnel, and experiments—to test new drugs so they can find more effective chemotherapies for breast cancer.

In Breastcancer.org, some members have researched the pharmaceutical industry and share with other members what they learn. Some members have investigated the role of pharmaceutical companies in the disease process of breast cancer, and they are frustrated about the financial commitments related to breast-cancer treatment and care for related side effects (like hormone imbalance and related complications). Much of their discourse includes references to the costs of treatments and the money that pharmaceutical companies gain by selling their products. For example, Marty twice references the cost for research—the first reference to pharmaceutical companies and the second to the Komen Foundation, which funds research into cures and treatments for breast cancer. Marty writes,

- "Wouldn't it be wonderful if iodine became a chemo that does not kill? Of course, the drug companies will fight it tooth and nail because they could lose billions."
- "As for Komen—all I can say is, after the millions and millions they have collected—Where is the damn Cure?"

In response to Marty, Gwenn shares her own opinion:

> Damn drug people. Take this one to fix what this one does to you & take this one to forget you are taking those two. That will be $1000.00 a month please. I quit.

Gwenn also shares information that she has read about the financial benefits for physicians who use particular drug:

> I also just read that doctors get a chemo bonus??? REALLY?? That is the most unethical thing I have EVER heard!

Marty does not provide reference information for her source; however, she seeks to connect with other members in her first reference by using a general third-person voice and by illustrating her emotion (her frustration) with multiple punctuation marks and capitalized letters in her second note about pharmaceuticals. In response, Maribeth writes,

> Chemo bonus??? WTH??? For God sakes. This makes me SICK!! I wonder if there is a friggin' RDS [Radiation Dosimetry Services] bonus too!!!

These women are frustrated by the financial cost to patients as well as the marketing structure that pharmaceutical companies have created to encourage physicians to use their products. The women posting these comments have finished most or all of their cancer treatments—they are discoursing about progesterone cream as a holistic treatment for their hormone issues after breast cancer—and so have experienced the high costs related to medical care for breast cancer. Their statements are responses to their experiences and the patient perspective that chemotherapy is expensive and that physicians should not be enticed by pharmaceutical companies to use certain chemotherapy drugs; physicians should prescribe those drugs that have been proven most effective.

In sharing their responses, the members express their anger and inform other patients of concerns about the costs of research and pharmaceutical drugs as well as the marketing structure for drugs, which seems unethical. (The ethics practiced by pharmaceutical companies is beyond the scope of this research, but company ethical standards are a concern, as outlined by Carlat [2013], who identifies issues in pharmaceutical ghostwriting, biased research and publications, data mining information about prescriptions, bonuses and gifts to practitioners, company-funded continuing medical education for physicians and speaking engagements by prominent providers.) These patients recognize some of the ethical dilemmas related to pharmaceutical companies and thus are logically considering situations that relate to them and sharing the logic with other members of the community. These women could increase their *ethos* if they provide information about *where* they hear these stories.

Discourse about pharmaceutical companies is minor compared to other medical topics. However, the references to these concerns are important because so many patients do undergo chemotherapy as part of their treatments and thus are a part of the pharmaceutical industry as consumers.

PATIENT DISCOURSE ABOUT HEALTHCARE PROVIDERS

In the data analyzed, patients most frequently reference their treatments when discussing elements of their experiences with the healthcare system.

They share details about their treatments as a part of their identity within the community and of their illness narratives. However, the second most frequent references to healthcare services are about patients' healthcare providers. Patients seek to communicate *with* their providers, but they also share with other patients what they experience when they interact with their providers. The healthcare provider is a patient's hope for truth, health, and a positive outcome. But when a patient's relationship with her provider is not positive, the patient may experience doubt, frustration, or distrust.

Patients need physicians. Physicians listen to their patients but also depend heavily on technology that provides diagnostic evidence to support what the patient reports (Levinson and Pizzo, 2011; Segal, 2005). "The patient's narrative itself [comes] to need translation—from patient's story to doctor's story. It . . . [needs] retelling in a way consistent with established medical knowledge" (Radin, 2006, p. 31). Patients, however, are rarely satisfied with passive involvement: many want to have access to information, including the results of their diagnostic tests, to participate more in their care (Samant, Aivas, Bourque, and Tucker, 2010; Shipman, 2010). They also want to know that their providers are well educated and are staying up-to-date on the newest developments in health and medical research.

Patients who communicate *with* their providers and participate in their own healthcare report a higher quality of life than those not involved (Kumar, Korthius, Saha, et al., 2010; Street and Voigt, 1997). Therefore, patients need to be encouraged to know more and say more, and they need to communicate with their providers—to take ownership of their health, to learn about their diagnoses and treatments, and to be involved in the decision-making processes. As patients are more a part of their care, they can provide feedback on their care and become more active agents of patient-centered change: "In the course of mutual support, it is only natural that some will identify targets for social action, from poor hospital procedures to environmental poisons. Thus, a community can, in its unstudied way, deal with issues of social policy (Radin, 2005, p. 592). And patients are identifying targets for social action as they discourse in online communities.

When patients feel unsure about their healthcare providers or about their relationship with the providers they may discourse with the other women in the community to find out how other patients are interacting with their providers and to gain advice on those patient–provider relationships. Many members in Breastcancer.org share their experiences with their providers; as consumers of healthcare services, patients consider their medical records, their experiences, and their outcomes as well as the care (paralleled sometimes to customer services and client satisfaction in the business model for medicine) that they receive. In response, they may express their agency—their logical considerations and decision-making processes related to their medical care.

Within the 469 posts that I analyzed, the women post 127 comments related to their healthcare providers. Of those, eighteen are positive and 109 are negative. The positive comments focus on physicians who listen to patients and consider the information that patients bring with them to consultations. The negative comments address patients' frustrations with their physicians not knowing about current research and treatment options or about communication issues that the patients have with their providers.

Those positive comments relate to open-minded providers. For example, Trish shares a positive note about her physician:

> Saw my wonderful, open-minded, up-on-just-about-everything PCP [primary care provider] (a board certified internist) today, and she was surprisingly negative about progesterone cream. I really need to study up on this now. . . She acted like it was a really bad idea, but she is open to any studies I can provide. . . . She reeled off a long list of very bad SEs [side effects] you can develop if you get too much progesterone, and also felt that there's not enough evidents that it's safe to do if you're PR+ [progesterone-receptor positive], as I am. . . . Anyway, I'm not deterred, but I really respect her, so it just means I'm going to have to read a lot more to decide if I want to go against her advisement.

Trish shares praise for her physician in her modifiers—"wonderful, open-minded, up-on-just-about-everything"—but her positive attitude about her physician is, according to the tenses and tone of her post, previously established. Trish expresses surprise to her provider's response and continues to express respect for her provider but contrasts that with her intention to research and to take new studies to her next appointment. In the end, Trish is going to decide what is best for herself by investigating the recent research on progesterone cream and, considering her physician's criticism of progesterone cream, she will come to her own conclusion.

Several members also express negative experiences and opinions of their healthcare providers. They criticize their providers' knowledge and consideration of alternative treatments, particularly related to natural and homeopathic treatments to their medical doctors. For example, Julia writes,

> Progesterone is surrounded by a profound lack of attention. I cringe when I see quotes like this from doctors "This is the only group of women at any age (bc [breast cancer] patients) that I advise to avoid using even low doses of transdermal progesterone or Prometrium capsules without consulting their oncologist beforehand. We simply don't know enough about the outcome either way." To my mind, this is a call to action, not a reason to stop testing for pr [progesterone] receptor status!

In her comment, Julia is subtly criticizing a physician whom Karen quotes in an earlier post; the physician states that the medical field does not know enough about progesterone treatments and their effects on breast-cancer patients to allow those patients to use those treatments. Julia disagrees with the physician, and she feels the freedom to voice her disagreement in her post and express her *logos* by explaining that, if the medical field does not know enough about a treatment, researchers should not stop testing but should increase testing until they have evidence for or against the treatment.

A few posts after Julia's statement, Kristi responds and addresses a difference between the information that the women are hearing from their providers and that they are finding in nontraditional research:

> All newly diagnosed patients are **overwhelmed** by information, particularly from the internet, and can't imagine how some of us "came up with" thinking that could possibly be so different than their oncologists or other docs.
>
> The answer is, we didn't "just come up with" a contrary perspective. We investigated long and hard and read the literature. **The doctors are not reading.** They are just following the official guidelines which are not evidence-based. The guidelines are consensus based. [Emphasis added.]

Kristi's response explains the logical, research-supported approach that the women in this community are taking to the alternative treatments they are asking about, trying, and suggesting to the other women who are interacting in this thread. Kristi questions the physicians' knowledge and thus their credibility by stating that they are not reading the research that the women on Breastcancer.org discussion board are reading.

Marty responds in kind, writing,

> The fact is we really do need to do our own homework because our doctors won't or don't have the time. They are sometimes the worst consumers. Since they are taught hours and hours by drug companies. They tend to believe they can solve everything with a pill. . . . How I wish I could get my doctors to open their minds. They are doing us all such a disservice.

Marty expresses a small amount of understanding—that physicians do not have time, and she understands that they will have limited information because they have limited time to investigate and read about new treatments. However, she finishes with a stronger tone, moving from the fact that they do not have or make time to read to the fact that physicians gain much of their continuing education and information about new pharmaceutical drugs from the companies that are researching, developing, and marketing those drugs. Her statement, "They tend to believe they can solve everything with a pill," shows that she believes the physicians are limited in their consideration of new therapies and treatments. And she finishes with a strong statement about her desire for her physicians to consider alternatives: "They are doing us all such a disservice." She unifies the community by including the other women—"us all"—and the other side of the issue, the physicians.

Several of the women state that patients need to educate themselves and not depend on what their physicians already know. As quoted earlier in this chapter, Kristi writes,

> We all have to read more than our doctors. Most of the time,when somebody comes back reporting what their doctor says, we find it's filled with holes and misinformation. The docs [doctors] are well-meaning but misguided.

Kristi challenges the other members of the committee to educate themselves; she insinuates that patients need to be prepared to suggest treatments and know what the current research reports, but she also justifies a patient's need to read with a physician's lack of knowledge. In this way, she creates a question about how prepared and up-to-date physicians are, stating (without evidence but with assuredness) that they mean well in treating patients but that they are not well prepared to consider the most current evidence. Her argument is weak, but because other community members agree with their statements about ill-prepared physicians, she aligns with other posts and thus builds on other members' arguments. In that way, she builds her *pathos* and *ethos* by agreeing with other members.

In the midst of this thread, Kristi shares that she has emailed the founder of Breastcancer.org and well-reputed oncologist Dr. Marisa Weisw, and then she criticizes Weiss's response to the email:

> If Dr. Weiss was really 'erring on the side of caution' she would READ the medical studies on progesterone before posting her personal theories and thoughts. The progesterone studies go back many years. There is no excuse for this kind of ignorance. Unless you are intimidated by going along with the standard-of-care medical community.

Kristi continues the argument that the other members are making—that healthcare providers do not approve of the most recent studies about progesterone cream—and resolves that providers do not approve because they do not know about the evidence for progesterone cream as a treatment for these women's hormone imbalances, and they do not know because they do not read; they are ignorant. She and several other posters also insinuate that physicians follow standard treatments to "go along with the standard-of-care."

Other members of the community share similar experiences. Sara reports that she asked her healthcare provider to help her with her hormones, reporting, "My doctors have so far offered no solution." Gwenn also reports her issues, reporting her provider's credentials but diminishing the oncologist's credibility:

> My first oncologist is the lead researcher on the bisphosphonates phase III trial at UAB [University of Alabama—Birmingham], among many other studies. She is suppose[d] to be one of the best breast cancer oncologists. UAB is one of the top Comprehensive Cancer Centers in the country. She had NO idea about the progesterone either.

Jamie continues by sharing her own experience and frustration:

> I asked the onco [oncologist] about DIM[2] —(my naturopathic doc strongly recommends it). The oncodoc never heard of it—I brought some info (from National Cancer Center or somewhere respectable) and had highlighted relevant stuff. He GLANCED at it and dismissed it. Said I should just eat some broccoli if I was concerned.

By discounting the research that Jamie has done and the information that she provided, the physician creates a separation between himself and his patients. And Jamie expresses her dissatisfaction with her physician's response by using all capital letters to emphasize the physician's response to the credible ("respectable," as she reports) source—"he GLANCED."

Gwenn states that she cannot trust a provider who lacks knowledge:

> My problem is that I have very little interest in what an onocologist has to say to me & IF he/she can't answer my questions why would I trust him/her? . . . I could give two rats butts about what any doctor's opinion. If I had listened to the last 8 I went to, I'd still have my tumor growing in my breast. They are human beings, they made mistakes.

Kate agrees by stating that she will continue to use progesterone cream and pay attention to the research because "the medical community DOES NOT KNOW how progesterone plays into our disease." (Several other members of the community share that they are using progesterone cream against their physicians' advice because the research they find supports progesterone cream as a therapeutic treatment.)

Julia builds *pathos* in the community by asking rhetorical questions to share her logic (building her *logos*):

> honestly, what would be the point in asking our oncologists about the wisdom of taking progesterone??? . . . they don't know any helpful answers. . . . And I'm supposed to seek guidance from a man who doesn't even bother to determine my menopausal status by looking at my estrogen levels as he writes out a refill for tamoxifen?

Julia concludes the discussion by summarizing what the members are asking: How can patients trust their healthcare providers if they find research that supports a treatment that is proven to help, and the trained professionals who serve as providers know nothing about it?

The members of the community use some effective rhetorical methods to express their frustrations and to reiterate their messages. Some of them use questions; they ask questions that have obvious answers. Other members use all capital letters to emphasize certain words in their posts; these words are meant to highlight the actions or characteristics that make the women question their providers' abilities to consider *all* of the available options and advise them per the most effective options. The women also post about their physicians' credentials, creating contrast between the physicians' qualifications and their lack of knowledge about diverse studies related to progesterone cream.

Physicians do have standards of care—regimens of care that have been established by controlled trials and evidence that supports the treatment that the physicians have established as the most effective—so studies that go against these standards may not be accepted by the community of healthcare providers within the medical community. But these patients criticize, creating a logical argument for the physicians' rejection of options and lack of knowledge about new treatments. By sharing their medical knowledge and criticizing their healthcare providers, these women empower themselves to control information and their circumstances and thus express their agency—their "capacity, condition, or state of acting or exerting power" (agency, n.d.). These comments acknowledge that healthcare providers are motivated to help patients but question the physicians' resources, schedules, and priorities. Part of this issue is that physicians commit to prioritizing their patients' needs (Moulton and King, 2010; Srinivasan, 2011), but they must provide healthcare to so many patients to meet their expenses and fund their salaries that they are limited in how much studying and reading they can do.

Other patients also share comments related to their providers. In the thread of posts titled "MPBC," six women post thirty-one times and share sixty-four references to their providers:

- providers in general (20 references),
- oncologists (10 references), and
- surgeons (9 references).

Three of the references are possessive—e.g., "my surgeon" (Katie) and "my doc" (Natalie). But these women, in the midst of their treatments, seem to respond more positively about some of their healthcare providers. For example, Katie states that, although the pathologist could not identify her cancer, her surgeon guessed correctly:

> so, i went nearly 2 weeks . . . because as my surgeon said, "your tissue has all the paths [pathologists] scratching their heads', basically saying' they didn't know what to make of it. . . . my surgeon kept telling them [pathologists] that she thought it was mpbc [metaplastic breast cancer]—she's only had 2 other cases with the same. and, when she called me with the results she said,' now don't go out there online and start reading about this because it will literally scare u out of ur mind. You need to wait to listen to and speak w/ the oncologist. . . . and, i proceeded to read, read, read and finally decided that it was too overwhelming and too scarey, just like she said.

Katie acknowledges that her surgeon was correct in the diagnosis and also in advising her not to research her cancer until she speaks with her oncologist. By stating, "just like she said," Katie builds her surgeon's credibility and affirms that her surgeon, having only seen two cases of metaplastic breast cancer, correctly determined the diagnosis. In her language, Katie divides the stakeholders in the situation into the surgeon, the pathologist, and herself.

In contrast, Lydia comments to establish her chemotherapy treatment as a team effort by stating, "It [catheter insertion] did get tough on my veins, but *we* were able to get one each time [emphasis added]." In separating the stakeholders, Katie gives her surgeon credit for correctly identifying her cancer and advising her correctly not to research, but in referencing herself as part of the actors, Lydia creates an air of collaboration related to her chemotherapy. Lydia later separates out the stakeholders, using a tone of passive compliance when she writes, "My onc [oncologist] is rather laid back about any testing, blood, or scans, which really bothered me at first. . . . but I'm slowly getting used to it now." Lydia chooses, for some reason, to accept the oncologist's preferences and practice habits and, in her statement, separates herself from the practitioner. The community members do not seem to agree on their roles and responsibilities related to care. As Lydia posts (mentioned above), she "gets used to" the physician's preferences and approach to practice. Another community member in this thread *asks* her provider about treatment; Mika writes, "but I'm going to talk to my onc [oncologist] about the change in the ER [estrogen receptor] if for no other reason then to put my mind to rest." Mika is also compliant but is less passive than Lydia; Mika will *ask* her physician about the treatment changes but not adapt or leave the decision-making to her provider.

In the thread of 176 posts from newly diagnosed members, the members refer to their providers:

- 56 references to surgeons,
- 49 references to physicians in general,
- 13 references to oncologists, and
- 8 references to primary care physicians.

Member state that they are going to consult a surgeon, that they have already met their surgeons, or that they do not like their surgeons. Newly diagnosed members are learning about their diagnoses, and they are searching for hope. They visit the community, seeking hope, but they also need hope from their providers. A lack of hope creates issues. For example, Emily reports,

> I was feeling so good that day *until* the phone call from my surgeon. He was very apologetic and supportive, telling me I had lots of options, etc. [emphasis added].

Several other newly diagnosed members report that their surgeons present options: Stephanie says, "We went to meet with surgeon was recommended and she told her [my sister] her options which was the lumpectomy or the mastectomy"; Lorraine reports that her mother's surgeon gave options for treatment; and Debbie and Kathy report that their surgeons have called. Cheri shares that her physician also called:

> I had my phone call last night from my surgeon who did a Lumpectomy 2 weeks ago. . . . He said that I should have a Sentinel node biopsy to see if the cancer has spread to the lymph notes, followed by a re-excision.

These members all share that their physicians communicate with them about their recommended treatments or the patients' options. They eliminate positive or negative tones and report fact about their interaction with their providers. The experienced members respond with advice: Becky advises, "do your research and make sure that you have a surgeon and oncologist that take time to answer all of the questions that you have," and Merlene suggests, "Once you have all this information, write down all your questions for you surgeon to answer." The newly diagnosed members and the respondents (and advisors) do not comment on positive or negative experiences with their providers. They simply state what they experienced and how they should prepare as they receive their diagnoses and treatment plans.

As the thread of posts grows, two members share in their introductions that they have issues with their surgeons' personalities, but both patients justify their choices to continue receiving care from those surgeons because of the providers' skills. Gayle writes,

> I actually went to my primary care dr. [doctor] on friday and asked him questions. my surgeon is supposed to be excellent but no bed side manor at all, no questions answered, he just looked at me like i should know what is next even though this is a first for me. the radiologist was very pleasant.

And Angie shares a similar situation:

> I do not like my surgeon but a friend said that she thought he had problems looking someone in the eye but as a surgeon she thought he would be ok.

Both newly diagnosed patients address their surgeons' personalities and compare that to the surgeons' skills, choosing surgical skills over "no bedside manner" and "problems looking someone in the eye." They use I-centered sentences to express their negative feelings but also giving evidence for why they do not like their surgeons. (Gayle does not give any feedback on her opinion about her primary care physician and does not support her feelings about her radiologist—"very pleasant"—with evidence. But both Gayle and Angie give evidence for their negative feelings.)

Experienced members encourage newly diagnosed patients to express their agency. Becky writes,

> Interview your potential doctors and if you don't like their "bedside manners" or the way that they deal with your questions, go see someone else for a second or third opinion. You are trusting these people with your life and health; trust has to be established first.

Becky uses second person to speak directly to the newly diagnosed patients; she does not use third person to give advice but moves to a personal tone to empower the newly diagnosed women in the community and to give them encouragement—even permission—to *choose* who provides their health care. And she brings up trust. The irony is that these new community members have not met her and do not know who she is; however, they trust her advice because she has breast cancer and has gone before them in the process. Therefore, she has already established her *pathos* because she can relate to what they are experiencing, her *ethos* because she is a member of the credible community of Breastcancer.org (and the newly diagnosed members are coming to join the community), and her *logos* because she provides a sensible justification for these new members to have a voice in their care.

Other threads also contain posts that justify patients getting second and third opinions. Stephanie states that she has met several surgeons who recommend different treatments and she asks, "How do you know who to trust?" Sophilia shares that three different radiologists read the same slides for her diagnostic testing and each has a different diagnosis for her disease. These patients include their agency, getting multiple opinions and diagnoses, as part of their illness narratives. However, they do not share details about their experiences, and they do not give their opinions about the providers who are giving them options or diagnoses. That void of the patients' opinions may be a symptom of their feelings as newly diagnosed patients, as those new members seem more unsure about their opinions and options than do the patients who are in the midst of or who are finished with their treatment for breast cancer.

Segal (2005) suggests that healthcare providers might separate themselves from their patients to objectively practice medicine. Frequently, medicine focuses on the provider's specialty and knowledge and the diagnosis and treatment rather than on the patient, who receives that care. Physicians and patients are separate because of their differences in knowledge, motivation, and investment in the situation; physicians train to treat breast cancer whereas patients are educating themselves (to a lesser extent than their physicians) to survive breast cancer and save their own lives. Therefore, patients are learning more and becoming a more active and more knowledgeable part of their own care:

> A kairology suggests that the symbolic moment of the credulous patient may also be passing, much like the symbolic moment of the stethoscope has, for the most part, passed. Direct-to-consumer advertising for prescription pharmaceuticals . . . disease support groups, childbirth and menopause movements, health information Web sites, popular pathographies, and patients' rights legislation are all part of a somewhat different rhetoric of patienthood. (Segal, 2005, p. 31)

Therefore, patients may separate themselves from practitioners who do not clearly explain the patients' diagnoses or treatments or if the patients do not trust the practitioner. This "rhetoric of patienthood" involves a patient's ability to know about her diagnosis and treatment and her feelings about expressing her illness narratives, including her experiences (Orgad, 2005). If a patient feels silenced or does not feel like she is part of the decision-making process, she will trust her physician less (Kraetschmer, Sharpe, Urowitz, and Deber, 2004). Patients trust when they perceive that their providers are comforting, caring, competent, and communicative (explaining *and* listening; Thom, 2001). Women also express more trust if their providers refer them to specialists and then check on their progress (Thom, 2001, p. 327). Although community members do not talk about referrals and check-ups in their discourse on Breastcancer.org, they do express preferences to physicians who listen to them, who have open minds, and who communicate. For example, Becky expands her agency and addresses trust and the patient's rights. (Portions of her posts have been presented earlier to make specific points, but the entire post reads as posted here.) Becky advises,

> After going through this the first time 13 years ago and now again, please take your time, do your research and make sure that you have a surgeon and oncologist that take time to answer all of the questions that you have. What was most important to me was ensuring that my doctors and I were in agreement with the treatment. . . . Interview your potential doctors and if you don't like their "bedside manners" or the way that they deal with your questions, go see someone else for a second or third opinion. You are trusting these people with your life and health; trust has to be established first. . . . Take the time to

> do your research, especially when dealing with the chemo drugs and their side effects. It really helps to have the knowledge before you get started. The drugs are definitely better than they were 13 years ago, and the side effects are treatable if you ask for help before you get started.

Becky encourages the other members to take control of their appointments and to ask questions because patients who do not connect with their physicians experience this separation. By using an imperative tone, she infers a personal second-person "you" to personalize her advice, but she also strengthens her tone by writing directly: "take your time," "do your research," "make sure," "interview," "go see someone else," and "take the time." Her imperative tone strengthens her advice, almost to instruction. Becky gives patients power by giving them direction.

When patients experience separation—either instigating it themselves or sensing it from their physicians—they may change physicians or they may approach other community members and ask for advice. Healthcare providers would be wise to listen to the discourse within these online communities to acknowledge these community members as humans and as agents of their own disease processes, to hear what patients are saying and sensing, and to identify ways that they can improve their skills related to how they relate to patients and to how they can eliminate this separation that patients can sense with their practitioners.

PATIENT DISCOURSE AND AGENCY IN THEIR NARRATIVES

Many patients struggle to exert their agency because they have no say about their diagnoses and thus feel powerless in choosing treatments. They may feel out of control in regard to decision making because they did not choose to have breast cancer or because they are not as knowledgeable as their physicians. Their agency—that is, their ability to sense any control or power over their circumstances, particularly over their treatment and recovery from breast cancer, and to act on that power—empowers patients to participate in the decision-making processes.

Agency is a point of contention between theorists—whether it is the ability or the intent for an individual to control the situation (Windsor, 2006).

> Agency on the surface seems like an uncomplicated concept—the individual ability to act, to choose[,] or to decide. However, the concept of individual action is caught up in a theoretical and philosophical controversy. The key binary terms in the debate are agency and structure. Agency refers to the capacity for freedom of action in the light of or despite social structures; structure refers to the social forces and constraints that affect so much of our social lives. (Schryer, Lingard, Spafford, and Garwood, 2003, p. 64)

In other words, agency describes an intention or behavior (Mooney and Ryan, 1993) but can also refer to a person's ability to act, regardless of the social norms that dictate what humans do. "Agency implies power" and relates to action (Giddens, 1984, p. 9); it does not require resistance to established leadership or authority but can describe one's ability to negotiate between conflicting views (Koerber, 2006) and to communicate an individual's options as well as the outcome of a negotiation (Campbell, 2005, p. 3).

As stated earlier, agency differs from structure, which identifies that different roles in the medical community have different purposes. Agency instead gives the patient the power to take her position in the medical community as the one who is receiving care. Applying agency, patients assert themselves when they participate in their medical decision-making, manage their own health, and participate in their care (Thomas, Aggleton, and Anderson, 2010), thus denying their patienthood (Tang and Anderson, 1999), which might require that they submit to the authority of a physician. "Agency offers hope for the alleviation of oppression through transforming the structural constraints imposed on people's lives" (Tang and Anderson, 1999, p. 86). Patients then must take authority in their medical care (Graham, 2009), which requires communication (O'Hair, Villagran, Wittenberg, et al., 2003). Agency frames patients' communication—as patients, as humans, as owners of their own bodies—and thus is an important element in analyzing patient-to-patient discourse about medical care.

In Breastcancer.org, members express their agency by posting in the community and by acting—by managing their care—in their consultations with their healthcare providers. They speak and tell their stories (Orgad, 2005; Pitts, 2004), they research, they establish their opinions, they make choices, they request second and third opinions, and they speak up. They also express their agency by posting in the community, also sharing their illness narratives and discoursing with other patients to build their stories and make decisions.

In particular, the members posting in the thread "Progesterone Cream" and suggesting nontraditional treatments for hormone imbalances assert their agency: they ask questions, gather information, and share in the responsibility of their medical care and decision-making (Segal, 2005, p. 35) by preparing resources to share with their healthcare providers. Some even choose to use progesterone cream, despite what their healthcare providers have told them. In this way, they challenge the traditional healthcare system and standard treatments by suggesting and testing homeopathic treatments. In this thread, Christine writes,

> If your Breast cancer was positive for hormones do not us nothing that have hormones can be even face creams, soy,etc, because it can trigger cancer again, I work in a cancer center and I see first hand the effect of creams,pills etc taken with no consultation with doctors; do not take herbs, teas, juices,

> creams without asking your oncologist;in the USA like many other countries there are no regulations , some herbs cancel the effects of some treatments, including birth control meds.

Christine seeks to build her credibility (*ethos*) by stating that she works in a cancer center and by affirming what some of members' medical doctors have told their patients. However, just as many of the other members have chosen to ignore their physicians' advice, they choose to ignore her advice. Several members are treating themselves by testing their hormones and using progesterone cream. Karen explains her logic for using progesterone cream:

> If cancer returns—new or recurrence—I don't imagine anyone is going to be able to tell me definitively it was this thing I did or didn't do that caused it. So I'm not going to beat myself up over having used the progesterone cream or not having done chemo or I ate too much birthday cake on my 50th. I'm going to live my life in a way that's fulfilling and meaningful to me, and if these "tools" help me do that for however long I have, then I'm good with it all.

Kate also asserts her agency by choosing what she will do with her body. She shares that she is using progesterone cream against her medical doctor's instructions:

> I don't know if I am right or wrong [about using progesterone cream] and I do know that compared to some of you I am not at as much of a risk (as compared to an individual here who might be dx'ed [diagnosed] at State II etc). Here's what I know. . . . So, for now, for me, I intend on continuing it's use. Until a doc [doctor] can fully explain to me what PR+ [progesterone-receptor positive] means I will continue to be on it [progesterone cream] for several years. . . . This is a very personal decision, and admittedly I have much less of a risk.. but that is the decision I have made until doc's have a better understanding of how progesterone works on an PR+ lesion.

Ruth states,

> I had experienced the typical SE's [side effects] and had sought medical support but received no more than a prescription for anxiety or told this is what I have to accept.CRAP I do, so I did my homework and decided to take Prog/Estrio/Test if it would help me have better quality of life.

Marty too expresses her agency and chooses how to act. She writes that she is waiting to start progesterone cream but she is monitoring her hormone levels. She posts,

> I guess I am being my own guinea pig, and I want to be able to have tests that prove how all these things are changing my numbers. This way, I can go back to my doctors and give them a piece of my mind, and see if I can get my

> insurance company to start considering these treatments. If we all do this, we may eventually have an influence on treatment protocols—at least we can pray we do. . . . It took a while, but change does happen. I believe we can make a difference.

Marty continues to express her agency in a later post:

> And do not feel like you are hopeless. It is a big overwhelming at first, but we have to really educate ourselves on all the options out there. We need to understand what protocols we follow so that we have faith in them. It may seem like a lot of work, which I guess it is, but it is really worth it. The more you learn, the more empowered you will feel, because you are making educated choices, that feel right for you, not just blindly following some doctors orders.

These women express their agency by gathering information but also by acting on the information they gather; as Marty explains, they make informed decisions for themselves (*logos*). These posts contain multiple references to "I"—a first-person emphasis that shows that each member is asserting herself and making her own decisions. These members understand and acknowledge that they may be risking their own health, but they are making choices to influence their own lives. They do not suggest that anyone else follow them, but they encourage other members to make their own decisions. Marty in particular diversifies how she expresses her agency. She advises and encourages other women, but she also tests her own hormones, considers using progesterone cream (against her physician's instructions), and anticipates that she will learn from her choices and perhaps advocate for other patients. In her discourse, the rhetoric of breast cancer includes agency—the action and motivation behind the words.

Agency allows patients to make choices about their own health care but it puts great responsibility on them to make decisions. For example, Cindy writes,

> [I am] leaning toward aggressive treatment. I will also second guess my decision if I do not. . . . it's a very personal decision and it really stinks when know one can tell you what to do, but keep pushing your doctors.

Nina also recognizes the power of her agency:

> I never realized how much control you need to take when dealing with breast cancer. So many decisions to make, and very scary because they [your decisions] are about your survival.

Terri asserts her agency by pursuing additional opinions. She writes,

> I have gone to a second opinion which the outcome is the same but her approach is different. . . . There are just so many options its all too confusing.

These women are expressing their agency by recognizing how frightening, overwhelming, and confusing the decision-making process is. The patients are not prepared to make decisions related to their care; they are expressing that they are unsure. But other members put their agency into action by choosing their treatments: Tracy shares, "I have chosen to remove both breast and have them reconstructed. I can't live my life worried about my other breast," and Laura also shares, "I have DCIS [Ductal Carcinoma *In Situ*] and have opted for a Surgical removal of both breasts." Tracy and Laura are acting on their agency and choosing additional treatment to control the situation and to eliminate risks of further cancer. In these five members' (Andy, Nina, Terri, Tracy, and Laura) statements on the discussion board, the women are discussing their agency using first-person and "I"-centric language, focusing on the members' feelings and choices. These women may not intentionally establish *pathos*, although many members would make these statements and choices, but they do logically (*logos*) explain why they are overwhelmed or why they chose elective mastectomies.

I end this chapter with Janie's statement:

> I refuse to let this cancer have power over me. I will not let it take me from my family. I will fight with all that I am and I do plan to win.

Janie does not waver in her agency or in her message: "I refuse. . . . I will not. . . . I will fight. . . . I do." Janie uses active, powerful language to assert her agency and to control what she can—specifically her response to the disease. She seeks to maintain some control. Many of the members in the community do seek control. They express their agency and thus they chose treatments, they research sources and information, they share their satisfaction and dissatisfaction, and they determine how they will respond to cancer. Unfortunately, when they assert their agency and speak decisively, they also disclose information and create privacy and confidentiality issues, which require that researchers consider the ethical dilemmas of studying patient-to-patient discourse (see chapter 4).

NOTES

1. Mika refers to her "adinum lab work," a term I have been unable to identify online, in medical dictionaries and textbooks, and through conversations with three physicians—a surgeon, a primary care physician, and an oncologist; therefore, I am unsure what laboratory works she is referencing in this post.
2. DIM is di-indoly methane, a plant-based dietary supplement that counters estrogen and helps normalize hormones (Lee, 2010). Dr. Lee addresses DIM on his naturalistic blog, citing thirty-six published sources as support for his description.

Chapter Four

Concerns Related to Privacy, Online Disclosure, and Ethics

When people communicate online, issues arise that relate to confidentiality, privacy, and disclosure. People share information with intended (primary) audiences but must also consider secondary and tertiary audiences. Their primary audiences are the receivers that they intend for their messages, but in public online spaces, other people may access their content. Those who are accessing this content should consider the ethical dilemmas related to using that information. For researchers, those ethical dilemmas include issues related to permissions, copyright, citations, and reporting research. These issues and considerations require that members of online communities as well as researchers consider the rhetorical situation, remember the humanity of those involved, and think ahead about consequences.

SELF-DISCLOSURE

When individuals interact in online communities, they choose what they discuss and disclose. This disclosure is not a problem as long as it is deserved and part of the relationship development; however, disclosure in a public place like a discussion board can be a risk for individuals who are sharing there because they may not realize they are being observed or that their personal information is available to more people than the intended audience. When individuals interact and share information about themselves, that information becomes co-owned by any parties involved in the interaction or by anyone who observes the interaction; all parties are then responsible for what they do with the information. However, these co-owners can include unintended audiences, such as lurkers (as referenced in chapter 1) who view the interaction but do not actively participate by reciprocating and sharing their own information.

Members who voluntarily share information expose a part of themselves; they self-disclose personal data. Self-disclosing is "the telling of the previously unknown so that it becomes shared knowledge" (Joinson and Paine, 2007). Self-disclosure is becoming a regular characteristic of discourse in online communities and is also creating issues in these online spaces. Self-disclosure is encouraged by emerging media and on social networking sites (Attrill and Jalil, 2011), such as Facebook (Butler, McCann, and Thomas, n.d.; Debatin, Lovejoy, Horn, and Hughes, 2009); Google (Rakower, 2011; Tene, 2008); blogs (Chen, 2012; Child, Pearson, and Petrionio, 2009; McCullagh, 2009); chat rooms (Yee and Bailenson, 2007; Zabinski, Celio, Jacobs, Manwaring, and Wilfley, 2003); and discussion boards (Kenen, Shapiro, Hantsoo, Friedman, and Coyne, 2007; Whilock, Powers, and Eckenrode, 2006). The social nature of these online spaces is relevant to online communities, because here, individuals become "members" and communicate and build relationships—actions that encourage and sometimes require the disclosure of personal information (Cate, 2010; Debatin, Lovejoy, Horn, and Hughes, 2009). Individuals may feel a sense of freedom in expression—because of their visual anonymity (Joinson, 2001) in a "faceless" situation and also in an effort to belong to a community by being similar through shared information.

Self-disclosure relates to the context in which the individuals are interacting (Antaki, Barnes, and Leudar, 2005), particularly in settings where they are likely to share personal information. That information is expected to be protected by both parties who are interacting. They may anticipate that they are sharing information that is private in a controlled environment. Online relationships encourage less guardedness but also allow for less control over information (Carter, 2004; Carter, 2005). What members forget is that membership in online communities is broad, and the members have no control over who is observing their interaction or taking ownership of their information. The Internet does not allow for the control that community members may anticipate; even if the community is password protected, the space can be hacked, posts can be copied, other members can share information, and users may not realize that others are present. Thus, as members disclose, they can create privacy issues as results of their intent, their identities, their trust, and their privacy (Attrill and Jalil, 2011; Ibrahim, 2008). "Hence the potential dangers and risks of willingly disclosing and displaying personal details become part of the architecture or code of these sites" (Ibrahim, 2008, p. 251). They can risk their security by exposing those personal details.

Online communities focused on medical diagnoses can create complex issues for members who self-disclose personal information. Members who share the details of their diseases put themselves at risk by exposing information that is considered personal or private. These community members typically share their illness narratives, which require a depth of disclosure related to the discloser's life, health, and medical information. For example, on Breastcancer.org, members must register to post on the discussion board and participate within the community. They join the community to interact and discourse with other members and to develop those relationships. However, Breastcancer.org's discussion board is public; the content is not password protected and anyone can read the content that members post in the discussion board. Breastcancer.org believes this is important for members to know; therefore, the Web page notes how many posts exist in a thread, but it also notes how many views the thread has (see figure 4.1.).

Online communities focused on personal and sensitive diseases like breast cancer create multiple dimensions of challenges as members self-disclose. Breast cancer is an intimate disease affecting a sexual organ that is equated to the identity of a woman. Men are also diagnosed with breast cancer, but for women, the amputation of the breast is the removal of part of her womanhood. Thus, when community members share information about breast cancer, their discourse can involve and encourage information that is more intimate than treatment of cancers that are internal, private, or removed with little external evidence of the treatment.

Because of the nature of online discourse and the intimate nature of breast cancer, members of online communities may share information that they

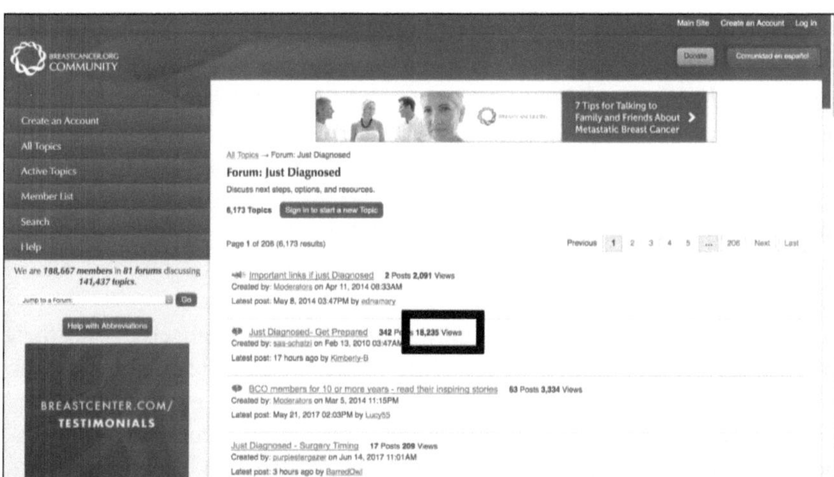

Figure 4.1. Screenshot from Breastcancer.org Community Page, Forum on Just Diagnosed that shows the titles of threads, the number of posts, and the number of views for the threads (boxed for emphasis).

would otherwise not share. They share intimate information about themselves online (Joinson, 2001; Joinson, 2004; Milson and Chu, 2002), as they discuss topics that might otherwise be considered inappropriate and that members later label inconsistent with their typical discourse. For example, in one post, one member shares her breast size while sharing her narrative and then writes, "I know, I know, TMI!!! I just need to spill my little heart out" (Jeanna). In another setting, her narrative including her breast size might have been judged inappropriate (and potentially embarrassing or sexually charged), but as women discuss the breast as the location of their cancer, they can share information about their breasts and consider that contextually appropriate. Other discourse is acceptable in the context of this online community. For example, members share personal experiences about hormone imbalance, which affects their sexual desires and causes side effects like hot flashes and vaginal dryness. Two members discuss their husbands' lack of libido, and the members reference their own libido eighteen times, sharing about their decreased libido before and increased libido after they use hormone cream (in the thread titled "Progesterone Cream"). Again, in other communities, such information might be inappropriate, but in this setting, the information is related to side effects of treatment for breast cancer that involves hormones.

Sharing, or "storytelling" (Orgad, 2005), is important as an individual moves through the process of expressing her agency: "Storytelling online is a potentially meaningful activity because it constitutes a way in which patients maintain and develop agency. That is, it is a process that enables patients to hold on to a sense of themselves as agents who have control, however little, over their lives" (p. 4). This storytelling is therapeutic (Beaudoin and Tao, 2007; Rodgers and Chen, 2005) and may be a coping mechanism as patients face their diagnoses. For these patients, "talk is both a prophylactic and a cure, offering a hopeful pathway towards happiness" (McLeod and Wright, 2009, p. 134). Therefore, as members "talk" and self-disclose, they benefit (Pennebaker, 1990; Pennebaker, 1993; Pennebaker, Kiecolt-Glaser, and Glaser, 1988; Pennebaker and Susman, 1988), and as they participate in the community, they benefit (Beaudoin and Tao, 2007; Rodgers and Chen, 2005).

As members of online community share, they put themselves and their personal information at risk, as their information can be obtained by anyone without accountability. Because they are focusing on other members, conversations, and the community members may not think about what they disclose. Membership begins this potentially risky process. When an individual decides to participate in Breastcancer.org, she registers and creates a profile so she can post on the discussion board, participate in the chat room, send personal messages, and join in the discourse that occurs in the online community. She creates a username, provides an email address, chooses a password, and agrees to the community rules. She can then edit her profile to add information that can include

- a photograph or avatar;
- demographic information such as her occupation, location, birthdate, and biographical information;
- forum-topic preferences; and
- disease-specific information.

She can also create a personalized signature that will attach to any post that she publishes. As members participate in the community and interact with other members, they slowly disclose information—their disease narratives but also information that could make their privacy vulnerable.

Members might expose information about their families, such as family support, which is an important element in a patient's well-being (Ballard-Reisch and Letner, 2003; Deshields, Rihanek, Potter, et al., 2012; Given, Given, and Kozachik, 2001; Gremore, Baucom, Porter, et al., 2011; Maly, Umezawa, Leake, and Silliman, 2005; Manne, Ostroff, Sherman, 2003; Rose, 1990). Family information is not public (although whitepages.com and similar pages now publish possible family links), but family information may include identifiers for the community members and their families that might not otherwise be publicly available. For example, on Breastcancer.org, members may post information about their families. (In the 176 posts in the "Just Diagnosed" thread, members share 59 references to their families.) Members may post about their children, an action that can conflict with the Children's Online Privacy Protection Act, or COPPA (Federal Trade Commission, 1998)—which protects children under thirteen years of age by protecting their personal information—and thus make their children vulnerable. For example, Gayle posts,

> i just want it gone so I can watch my 4 children grow and grow some more

and Linda shares,

> [I] have two wonderful young kid's who need me their only 10 and 14!!!

These members may share about family as their source of support, but they may also share because they are concerned about their ability to battle cancer and still care for their families (Ashing-Giwa and Lim, 2010). For example, Susan shares,

> I care for a mentally ill father and aunt with depression who is older. . . . I am divorced, no siblings, no children, no contact with my natural mother.

As they share, they may be sharing about their greatest joy or their greatest responsibility and how it will be a part of their disease narrative.

Members' disclosure of family information is an important element related to the rhetoric of breast cancer. Members' posts typically relate to how breast cancer will affect their families, including their children. The member shares specifics that help to build *pathos* because she is talking about her role, for example as mother, and her inability to care for her children during the disease process, and many members struggle with taking care of their families during their care. Even in "Just Diagnosed" threads, newly diagnosed members anticipate that they will struggle because they logically consider the side effects of their treatments and the energy and time that their families need as well as the amount of care they as patients will need as they confront breast cancer.

Equally private and a source of frustration is a lack of support, and members may share this as well. Family may not be able to cope with breast cancer—with the unknown, with the potential outcome of cancer, with a lack of control, and with other challenges. Community members may share this private information and discuss a sometimes lack of support, such as Alicia's post:

> I, too, was diagnosed this week. . . . I have cried the past 2 days, and this site has helped me as well. I am not getting much support from my spouse at the moment.

In response, Adrian (a member for 5 years and author of more than 8,000 posts) responds:

> Husbands arn't a lot of help at first, too much shock, I guess. . . . Tell your husband what you need, he hasn't a clue and there is a good book for him.

Then Ava, a new member (of less than 1 month), interjects,

> I'm sorry you aren't getting much support from your spouse. Maybe it is just that he's still shocked too. I'm so sorry you are having to go through this. . . . PM [personal message] me anytime . . . if you want to talk.

These members discuss a lack of support, a topic that is minimally researched (Manne, Ostroff, Sherman, et al., 2003). The existing research illustrates that family is valuable in a patient's coping with stressors related to breast cancer; thus, this valuable element of their disease narrative would be obvious information for them to disclose as they create relationships with other members in the online community. By sharing their struggles during their treatments and the perceived or real lack of support, members in the community are seeking empathy from other community members. They belong because they share the diagnosis of breast cancer, but they build their *pathos* by sharing their struggles of having little or no support.

Community members may also disclose their location—a country, a state, a city, and additional information that they may share in their posts. Location on its own may not serve as an identifier—information that allows someone to determine an individual's identity—but if it is combined with other information, location can point to a woman's identity and void her anonymity and privacy in a public online community. One thread focuses on location as women ask if other members live in their regions (of the United States and the world) and as they announce face-to-face gatherings. In this thread, women openly discuss their locations and plans to meet at a geographic location. But throughout their posts and profiles, members may expose information that identifies their locations; they may not need to be as specific as pinpointing an event they are attending. For example, in the thread called "Progesterone Cream," forty-eight women post; of those posts, twenty-seven (56.3 percent) include a state, a city and state, or a country outside the United States in the discourse within the posts. And, whereas some of the members do not openly state their locations, two posts include a reference to location in their usernames, and several others note some grocery store or physician in a location in a city. The diversity of members' locations supports that these relationships are strongly established in this online community—shared locations vary from the United Kingdom, Canada, and fifteen states (as far northeast as MA and as far northwest as WA)—despite the members' geographic distance. However, including locations also adds to the risks of the members' privacy.

As the women discourse, they share more and more information—about their opinions on the healthcare system, about challenges with insurance, about political preferences, and other information that indirectly may relate to their illness narratives but that also exposes more information about who they are. As they post, some of the members drop usernames and begin to refer to others by their first names. For example, in the "MPBC" thread, Elisabeth writes,

> i notice that some gals put their names at the end of comments, others just their call letters, etc. my name [. . .] is sometimes shortened to [. . .] by others & it's easier to keystroke—but the easiest is [. . .] and i'm all for easy . . . so, is there really a preference among these threads or just left to the individual?

Lydia responds,

> Some women don't ever put their real names out there. . . . I like knowing names, I think it's nicer that way. ☺

She later shares,

> If anyone here is on Facebook, 'friend' me, I am [. . .] on FB.[1]

In posts, these women may also include their ages and information about their professions.

Some community members may be concerned about posting their private information (Swenson, Constantinides, and Gurak, 2002, p. 342), but others may not recognize the issues that self-disclosed information can create. They may focus on belonging in the community and on building their *logos*, *ethos*, and *pathos* rather than considering that each bit of data is out of their control when they expose information in a public community and that others with no virtue can piece those bits together (like a puzzle) to create a profile and falsely represent that member. This type of crime is not frequently addressed, and community members may not be aware; they may not recognize danger when they publish private information in a public community. However, in a time when cybercrime is a daily concern—so much so that the U.S. government's Federal Bureau of Investigation (FBI) focuses on online crimes (Federal Bureau of Investigation, n.d.)—individuals need to beware of the information they share online.

PRIVACY AND HIPAA

In considering self-disclosure in public online communities, most disconcerting is the members' sharing their medical information and posting their medically focused signatures. When they register for the community on Breastcancer.org, they can share their medical history and they can create signatures that are automatically attached to each post and thus are published throughout the community's text. This disclosure of medical information is an extreme example of the self-disclosure occurring in the online community, because some of the posts and signatures include medical information that is legally protected by HIPAA.

HIPAA—the Health Insurance Portability and Accountability Act—was enacted in 1996 by the U.S. government to respond to growing concerns about how to protect citizens' private medical information (DHHS, 2003). The act protects workers' insurance when they change jobs and also creates standards for the transferal and storage of health data in medical records and billing information. When information is transferred, privacy becomes a concern. HIPAA includes a "Security Rule" and a "Privacy Rule" that outline standards to protect patient privacy (DHHS, 2003)—as physicians, other providers, and insurance companies use, transfer, store, and disclose "protected health information."

> A major goal of the Privacy Rule is to assure that individuals' health information is properly protected while allowing the flow of health information

> needed to provide and promote high quality health care and to protect the public's health and well being. (p. 1)

HIPAA also outlines how to instruct patients about their privacy rights and how providers and insurance companies can use medical information (Berle, 2011; Hader and Brown, 2010). It also identifies certain information as "individually identifiable health information" that must be protected. This identifiable information

> is information, including demographic data, that relates to:
>
> - the individual's past, present or future physical or mental health or condition,
> - the provision of health care to the individual, or
> - the past, present, or future payment for the provision of health care to the individual
> - and that identifies the individual or for which there is a reasonable basis to believe can be used to identify the individual (DHHS, 2003, p. 4).

In other words, information that can be used to identify or inhibit care for an individual (e.g., financial history) is not to be released by healthcare organizations (e.g., insurers, providers, and clearinghouses; pp. 2–3). These organizations are working to comply with HIPAA (Blobel, 2011; Birnhack and Elkin-Koren, 2011) and not be penalized with fines, closures, and legal action. The responsibility for privacy outlined in HIPAA focuses on those who handle health data (Adesina, Agbele, Februarie, Abidoye, and Nyongesa, 2011; Anton, Breaux, Gritzalis, and Mylopoulos, 2011). This act ensures that a patient's medical information is secure because this information—about genetics, diagnoses, testing, appointments, medical treatments, etc.—can influence others and create bias that may influence decisions related to a patient's insurance or employment. However, individuals can disclose their own information; if they do, they should know that they may create issues related to their own privacy.

In their posts, online community members may disclose data about their medical histories, diagnoses, complications, family histories, treatments, and other information in their posts. They may include other medical information as well. For example, Susan writes,

> I suffer from chemical depression, bipoloar type II and OCD [obsessive compulsive disorder]. . . . I have back problems and am awaiting a disability hearing in 00–00 0000 for my back and mental chemical imbalances. . . . I am divorced, no siblings, no children, no contact with my natural mother- that is not even an option-and I am frightened and depressed.

Another member, Margaret, joins in and shares protected medical information:

> I finally started taking a low dose of Paxil. That helped. . . . I can relax and not have panick attacks.

And a third member, Melissa, shares her family history as well as her current diagnoses in detail in her post:

> I'm 50, just underwent a total abdominal hysterectomy 8 weeks ago, they thought I had ovarian cancer. Everything came back negative and what they thought were tumors, were fibroids. I am also having some concerns with my bowels. I've had IBS [irritable bowel syndrome] for years, but am having some blood there. I also have Lupus, and Fibromyalgia. I'm not in the greatest of shape physically, am overweight, but don't have much energy for exercise. I also am anemic have been for years, so that's another concern. My grandmother and her mother both had breast cancer, a cousin had the exact same type I have at about 37, had a dual mastectomy and has been cancer free for 17 years. . . . My father died of lung cancer, but it had reached the lymph nodes and spread all over his body before they caught it. It was very aggressive.

These three members share HIPAA-protected information; however, they do not expose their names, locations, or other information that might allow a deviant "visitor" to the community to identify them. In this way, they rhetorically act on their *ethos* as members of the community for patients diagnosed with breast cancer but also share their *logos* by justifying the information they are sharing and their *pathos* by seeking to share information that affects other members to sympathize or empathize with them.

In contrast to these posts of private medical information with no identifiers, signatures can contain information that can identify a patient. (I have substituted information in the sample signatures to protect the women who have used these signatures.[2]) For example, Lois' signature provides incredible detail after she includes her location after her username at the top of her post. Her signature reads,

> Lois–age 44, IDC & ILC ,Rt. Mastectomy 00/00, 0/0 nodes,1.1 cm & 1 cm, stage 2, gr. 3, ER+/PR+, Her2NU+++, TCH chemo 00/00–00/00, Herceptin through Dec. 00 T.E.@ mast. Surgery, silicone implant exchange January 0000, allergic to Tamoxifen

In this signature, Lois includes

- her diagnoses with types of breast cancer (invasive lobular breast cancer [ILC] and invasive ductal breast cancer [IDC]);
- the surgical treatment (mastectomy of right breast) and date of treatment;

- the number of nodes that are cancer positive;
- the size, stage, and grade of the tumors;
- her hormone-receptor status;
- her chemotherapy and hormone-receptor treatments and dates of treatment;
- her reconstruction method and date; and
- her related drug allergies.

This information documented by a physician or insurance company is HIPAA protected; however, the community member can disclose this information with no protection or penalty, and every time she posts, she increases the probability that the information will be seen by visitors.

Another example comes from Carolyn, who is one of the most frequent participants. She signs her posts

> DX 0-00-00 IDC 1.1cm Stage 1 Grade 2 SNB 0/5 ER+ PR+ HER– Bi-Lat Mas re-con,tissue expanders on 00/00—Exchange to silicone implants on 00/00/00 Oncotype DX Score 9. . . . If God brings you to it, he will get you through it

Similarly, Carolyn exposes information that is HIPAA protected and that provides medical identifiers. Paired with personal information that she discloses in her posts, this information can increase Carolyn's vulnerability per her privacy and security. In this signature, Carolyn includes

- her date of diagnosis;
- her diagnosis with type of breast cancer (invasive ductal breast cancer [IDC] with notations about estrogen and progesterone receptor status);
- the size, stage, and grade of the tumor;
- the number of nodes (SNB—sentinel node biopsy) that are cancer positive;
- the surgical treatment (bi-lateral mastectomy with tissue expanders to prepare for reconstruction) and date of surgical treatment;
- her reconstruction method (exchange from expanders to silicone implants) and date;
- her oncotype diagnosis score, which indicates how her genetic makeup will respond to the cancer; and
- a personal quote that gives her hope.

A third example (for Lydia) includes similar medical information—

> Diagnosis: 00/00/0000, DCIX, <1cm, Stage 0, Grade 2, 0.0 nodes
> Diagnosis: 00/00/0000, IDC, 2cm, Stage IIa, Grade 3, 0/6 nodes, ER-, PR-, HER2-

Within her previous discourse in the thread, Lydia also provides her first name, her location, and her children's ages. Paired with her medical history, identifiers, and information that makes her security vulnerable, this information endangers the community members' privacy and her identity. In this signature, Lydia shares

- her first diagnosis, which includes
  - her diagnosis date and cancer type (probably a typographical error, as Ductal Carcinoma *In Situ* [DCIS] is a typical cancer type);
  - the size, stage, and grade of the tumor;
  - the number of nodes (SNB—sentinel node biopsy) that are cancer positive; and
- her second diagnosis date (four years later), which includes
  - her diagnosis date and cancer type (and invasive ductal breast cancer [IDC]);
  - the size, stage, and grade of the tumor;
  - the number of nodes (SNB—sentinel node biopsy) that are cancer positive; and
  - notations about estrogen and progesterone receptor status.

Lydia has been a part of the community of breast-cancer patients for two rounds of the disease. Thus, she builds her *ethos* within the community by having gone through one round of the disease process and returning for her second round. She also is a member who readily shares personal information, creating relationships and comfortably interacting with the other members. She establishes her *pathos* easily with her participation in the community: no one would choose to be a member of this "club," and no one would *ever* choose to be a second-time member.

A majority of women in the community include some automatic signature. Not all signatures are as detailed as those addressed above; some are simplified to one line and emoticons, such as Karen's signature—

> dx ICD er+ pr+ stage1 grade2 node-her2- 3.2cm M !!!

and Brenna's signature—

> Dx 00/00/0000, LCIS, 3 cm, Stage II.

However, these signatures still contain information that makes the members vulnerable. They include information about their diagnoses and, with the information the members may share in their posts, they increase their vulnerability.

Posting this information helps community members belong in the community—they share information and diagnoses with other community members and thus build their *logos* (I am here because I have breast cancer.), their *ethos* (I am a member because I too have breast cancer.), and their *pathos* (I am sharing my disease here, where others understand.). Posting also helps members feel in-control of their medical information and become empowered to share information when they choose. By controlling this information, they express their agency. However, they also share in a public community that allows anyone who has Internet access to obtain their information and become co-owners of these members' valuable medical information. For them, the line between public and private may seem less clear in online communities (Beddows, 2008; Kastman and Gurak, 1999). But the reality is that information on the Internet is accessible (Costigan, 1999)—by those maintaining the server, those registered to access the community's content, and those who have access to information in public spaces. Members of these online communities need to recognize the risks they take when they share their medical information and other identifiers in public online spaces.

ETHICAL CONCERNS: COPYRIGHT, CITATIONS, AND REPORTING RESEARCH

One of the unintended audiences of posts in public communities may be researchers who gather information in online spaces. They assess online practices of community members and use that information to predict online behavior, to better understand members in these communities, and to create better online tools. Researchers need to be aware of ethical research standards and should be focused on the people involved and then on the research they are analyzing. Ethical research and reporting requires that the researcher considers the writers of online artifacts, the purpose of the online community, and potential consequences of studying the community and reporting findings as well as the researcher's responsibilities to cite others' intellectual property.

Researchers' understanding of ethics is part of their fields' identities (McBride, 2005, p. 2), and although scholars have borrowed many ethical standards, the rhetoric of health and medicine is seeking to establish its own standards of ethics. This study also seeks to continue this pursuit of these standards. Our ethical standards require a variety of priorities and values. The ethic of virtue, introduced by Aristotle, establishes that an individual should control himself and choose to act with good in mind, seeking to do that which is virtuous and excellent (Aristotle, n.d./350 BCE.); this ethic focuses on the motive and character of the actor. A Kantian ethic, named after Immanuel Kant, challenges the individual to not harm any other creature, providing an absolute moral law that states that the actor must consider the outcome or consequences of the action to ensure that no one is harmed (Johnson and Cureton, 2017). A utilitarian ethic, combined from the writings of several philosophers (most known are Jeremy Bentham and John Stuart Mill; Singer, 2003), focuses on the best outcome for the largest number of stakeholders and thus requires the actor to responsibly consider the direct and indirect consequences of the decision being made. The ethics of care is a relational ethic that requires that the actor listen, interact, and act according to the best outcome for those who are closest to the actor (Noddings, 2012). A variety of other ethical theories exist, depending on the desired outcome and priorities of the decision maker. (This topic is too broad for a full description of ethical theories that apply; however, I have chosen the most frequently used in ethical studies.)

The ethical researcher is seeking information with a utilitarian purpose—to ensure the greatest good for the most number of people; however, the online researcher also needs to apply a Kantian philosophy to do no harm to those who are interacting in the online space and to choose methods of research and reporting that benefit the most people but that also minimizes—preferably alleviates—all inconvenience, discomfort, or harm to others. Ideally, the research will not harm any of the community members but will benefit (now and in the future) all community members, researchers, and designers as well as secondary stakeholders such as family members, information architects, communication theorists, and other scholars and researchers. The online researcher can seek to be ethical by submitting a research protocol to the IRB and thus be accountable for ethical research design and implementation of the project. As stated earlier, IRB applications can create challenges for researchers (King, Bivens, Pumroy, Rauch, and Koerber, 2017) because applications typically focus on the researchers' ethical responsibilities as they gather data directly from human subjects and request information about gathering data from already existing artifacts, such as medical records and established databases. In approving applications for research, the IRB wants to ensure that the researcher considers the potential risks that human subjects may experience in participating in the project; thus, the IRB expects the researchers to inform human subjects of the time and commitment they will invest in data collection and to explain the potential risks that subjects might face, such as pain or emotional distress. The IRB also ensures that subjects' rights are protected and that subjects can leave a study at any time. The IRB application may not specifically ask about the overlap between artifacts and the humans that created the artifacts; the standards address traditional texts such as medical records, databases, and pre-existing documents rather than organic documents that change daily—that are being built by and around individuals in a living, breathing online community. Thus, researchers should submit themselves to their review boards but should understand that each research project has unique characteristics, specialized questions, and potential complications.

When researching online artifacts, researchers must carefully report those artifacts as the creators' intellectual property that is protected by law (McKee and Porter, 2009, p. 53); a researcher cannot claim the artifacts as their own creations. However, giving credit to the creator creates a conflict between privacy and citation and between protection and credit. Intellectual property includes written data and media such as online texts, images, and audio and video files. U.S. law requires that, when using (or reproducing) a portion of another person's intellectual property, the researcher must cite the source. Reproduction is simple because so much intellectual property is not digitized and can be gathered and easily reproduced. The law says to cite but does not dictate a style or the information required in the citation. In citing, the researcher must consider if ethical reporting means citing full sources, which denies privacy and thus may damage the humanity of women through the content where community members express agency in the context of an online conversation. These members deserve protection to ensure that their texts are exposed as little as possible to unintended audiences. ("Unintended audiences" are audiences that the author did not originally consider or that may be indirectly and accidentally driven to the texts by other means, such as researchers' reports of their findings.)

Elm (2009) writes, "When we ensure that our research subjects are not harmed, humiliated, or offended, it may not always be necessary to follow single rules and regulations exactly" (p. 85). Elm is suggesting that, in seeking to ensure that research is ethical, researchers may be able to alter rules to ensure that the humans involved are unharmed. This theory also aligns with the lack of citation standards in the law and thus enables the researcher to determine what information is necessary to ensure that the citation style is legal and ethical.

For online discourse, a fine balance exists between researching publicly published texts and protecting the origin of a text; that balance involves not only harming members and creating negative consequences for the community as a whole but also to protecting personal and sensitive information. Therefore, sources of quotes should not be identified fully if identification creates potential harm for the community and its members and if identification could drive unintended audiences to community-members' posts. In researching a medically focused community, the researcher needs to consider even more issues related to the community. If a researcher cites the sources of quotes from individual posts from patients, that researcher potentially exposes a patient's illness narrative, conversation, signature, and profile (any of which may contain HIPAA-protected information) to unintended audiences that could cause harm to the patient. Therefore, to protect the integrity of the community from research outcome, texts should be identified as someone's intellectual property but should not be cited per standard citations.

For my study and for the posts included in this report, I choose quotes that do not contain sensitive, personal, or protected information but instead paraphrase those quotes to protect the content of a quote that might be found via search engine and the Internet. All posts that are quoted are quoted as the community member wrote; irregular spacing and creative spelling, punctuation, and grammar are included as in the original post to illustrate and respect the author's emotions, voice, and expression. Therefore, quotes are authentic and sensitive content is paraphrased to protect the context of the individual's post without driving an unintended audience to sensitive posts. (This practice aligns with methods of other respected researchers, such as Bodle, 2011; Kastman and Gurak, 1999; Gallagher, 2009; Orgad, 2005; Radin, 2006; Sidler and Jones, 2009; Still, 2008.)

Citation also creates a challenge; a typical citation for an online post includes the community member's name (or username, if the writer has created one); the title and date of the post; and a URL. This citation then enables the audience to visit the original source. Citations exist for three purposes: to give the originator credit for the intellectual property, to build the credibility of the person who is citing the original intellectual property, and to provide the audience with the original source for additional research on the topic. This third purpose is the most difficult in ethical analyses, because the audience may not be potential members of the community. By including a Web address (URL), the citation can drive an unintended audience to the community and to the specific post. Although the post is publicly published and thus accessible to anyone with Internet access, the writer's intent is rarely to publicly express the post content or to bring crowds to the community site. Therefore, for this study, texts are identified and credited double-blinded pseudonyms for the community members' usernames and Web addresses for the original posts are omitted. (The community's Web address is the only one included.) This system protects the members and their privacy but, as stated earlier, identifies that a post is not my intellectual property. I credit the community—in this project, Breastcancer.org—and therefore create a standard citation style by using in-text or parenthetical notations with the community member's assigned pseudonym. (All citations from sources outside the posts on Breastcancer.org follow standard citation style of the American Psychological Association.) Through this citation method, members' voices are presented in context and the integrity of the narrative in the posts and the context of the thread are maintained but ethically protected.

In this research, I make additional efforts to protect the community members and their identities. First, I respect the virtual identities of the community members of Breastcancer.org and take pains to ensure that I am unable to identify any of the members. I do not visit community members' profiles or gather identifiers to search for them in other threads on Breastcancer.org, in other online communities, or in the white pages or other databases that provide information for tracking individuals: to do so would be to violate the community members' privacy. Second, by citing posts with a pseudonym for the community members' username, I ensure that unintended audiences cannot track individuals from the narrative that I include in my research findings.

Researchers must make ethical decisions related to the methods they are using for their investigations. Because ethnographers are studying (and thus experiencing) a culture, an ethnographer may participate in that culture. However, in an online community, the ethnographer brings personal biases as well as research objectives; therefore, for virtual ethnographies, the researcher should observe and document but should not influence the culture—or the voices of the community members—with her own words. (For this study, I chose not to participate but to observe. I registered for Breastcancer.org and posted twice in 2008 and then withdrew. Two years later, I chose to observe the culture within Breastcancer.org, so I designed this study, obtained IRB approval, and began to gather data. However, I decided to continue to not participate because I did not want to be considered a troll, to disrupt the community members' interaction, or to prompt any narrative in a thread but rather to allow the interaction between members to develop organically.) To conduct ethnography, an individual applies for review-board approval; therefore, to conduct a virtual ethnography, the researcher should also apply for approval, even though the data set will consist of artifacts. In studying publicly accessible artifacts, some researchers believe that research consent is automatic (Whitty and Joinson, 2009; Young, 2001); Breastcancer.org (n.d.) agrees, informing community members that anyone may access the community. Other researchers believe that members of online communities consider their posts to be personal (Im, Chee, Lim, et al., 2007; McKee and Porter, 2009; Owen, Bantum, and Galant, 2009; Whitty and Joinson, 2009); therefore, researchers need to maintain an ethical do-no-harm mindset (McKee and Porter, 2008, p. 738). For this study, I recognize that online discourse in a medically focused community contains sensitive and HIPAA-protected information, such as demographic and diagnoses-specific data; therefore, I use only publicly accessed artifacts and blind the community-members' pseudonyms (as did Still, 2008). This method of reporting also is consistent with standard established in the Belmont Report, which protects human's rights in research (OHSR, n.d.).

NOTES

1. I have omitted the members' names to protect their identities, but they do not take the same precautions.

2. I have changed dates in posts to 00/00/0000 (or a format similar to the original content) to protect the creators of the posts, as diagnoses, treatment, reconstruction, and appointment dates may be identifying information.

Chapter Five

Big Data and the Rhetorics of Health and Medicine

Medicine rotates around information: about disease, patients, drug interactions, new developments and equipment, effective practice, healthcare policies, and a myriad of other datasets that affect the delivery of care and patient health. Without this information, healthcare professionals cannot diagnose disease, prescribe treatments, or predict potential outcomes. The patient is the primary source of information, providing details about symptoms, illness narratives, and the vessel in which the disease exists; the patient is central in the disease process and thus in the field of medicine.

Patient privacy is of the utmost importance. U.S. legislation protects patient information through HIPAA, requiring high levels of standardization and privacy in the transmission of information between practitioners, referring physicians, healthcare support, hospitals, electronic medical records (EMRs), and insurance companies or governmental agencies that supplement coverage funding. (See chapter 4 for more information about HIPPA.) Patients are required to sign consent and awareness forms to verify that they understand the restrictions on information transferal and that they release their practitioners to discuss their medical records with other physicians, insurance companies, and family members. The restrictions are necessary to ensure patient privacy, but the standardization of privacy protection has created challenges for providers who seek information about the current medical trends. To predict trends, researchers and analysts are now gathering blinded data in massive amounts to analyze without identifying individual patients. The amount of data is overwhelming.

This chapter briefly introduces the future of online data and then turns that discussion to address how patient discourse and the rhetorics of health and medicine might be affected by big data. Online information is already being mined to determine statistical analytics and trends, and organizations in every industry are analyzing mined data to create profiles of the individuals who use those industries.

BIG DATA AND DATA MINING

Big data is a growing industry that involves the management of large amounts of otherwise unmanageable bodies of data and thus provides any industry with a competitive edge because the data provides real-life information on members of the potential market for that industry. Big data involves complex processes because of the amount of information that technology is gathering and storing. Capturing, or *mining*, that data allows corporations to learn about their potential markets from the market and its members' behaviors in real life. "Data mining is the extraction of hidden predictive information and unknown data, patterns, relationships and knowledge by exploring the large data sets which are difficult to find and detect with traditional statistical methods" (Kaur and Bawa, 2015). However, big data involves more than just data mining. Once the data is captured, it is stored in large databases that allow researchers to analyze, query, and curate the data. To analyze the information gathered, *data scientists*[1] manipulate the data to obtain knowledge about large-scale trends and to predict behavior and outcomes. The amount of data is too large for humans to manage without the benefits of technology: e.g., "IBM estimates that we are generating 2.5 quintillion bytes of data each day, more than 90 percent of which was created in the last 2 years" (Silver, 2012). (That amount—2.5 quintillion bytes—of data equals 2,500,000,000,000,000,000 bytes of data, which "would fill 10 million blu-ray discs, the height of which stacked, would measure the height of 4 Eiffel Towers on top of one another" [Walker, 2015]. To consider units of data, see table 5.1.) The amount of data is overwhelming, and humans around the earth continue to create data. For example, in each *minute* of 2015, we

- uploaded 72 hours of YouTube videos,
- Tweeted 277,000 Tweets,
- published 216,000 Instagram posts, and
- sent 204,000,000 emails (Walker, 2015).

Of the data humans create, 90 percent is unstructured (Walker, 2015), which means that it is submitted in small units of communication—such as logs, emails, calls, and photographs—but does not exist in a way that it can be analyzed and interpreted to predict large-scale trends. Analysis and interpretation requires trained individuals to create and use data management systems. IBM (n.d.a.) predicts that 4.4 million data scientists will be necessary to handle the amount of data already collected, and because that amount of data is increasing daily, the number of data scientists needed will only increase.

Data is stored in large databases that can hold the data until they are needed, transferred, or sold to other corporations that manipulate the data to determine trends in large samples. "Big data is changing the way people within organization work together. It is creating a culture in which business and IT leaders must join forces to realize value from all data" (IBM, n.d.a.). Organizations cannot underestimate that, by analyzing data from a potential market, audience, or clientele, they can better anticipate customers' preferences, needs, and expectations.

Big data exists everywhere, and frequently, that data is free and readily available: through repositories that already exist, including data.gov, the U.S. Census Bureau, Facebook Graph, Google Trends, and Amazon Web Services public datasets (Marr, 2014). The data is manipulated through software created to statistically analyze unimaginable amounts of data, identifying variables and correlations in populations that previously were too large to consider.

Table 5.1. Current Measurements for Data Storage*

Unit of Measurement	*Abbreviation*	*Value Related to Bytes*	*Size of Unit in Bytes*
bit	b	0 or 1 bit**	1/8B
byte	B	8 bits**	1B
kilobyte	KB	1000^1B	1000B
megabyte	MB	1000^2B	1,000,000B
gigabyte	GB	1000^3B	1,000,000,000B
terabyte	TB	1000^4B	1,000,000,000,000B
petabyte	PB	1000^5B	1,000,000,000,000,000B
exabyte	EB	1000^6B	1,000,000,000,000,000,000B
zettabyte	ZB	1000^7B	1,000,000,000,000,000,000,000B
yottabyte	YB	1000^8B	1,000,000,000,000,000,000,000,000B

* Adapted from "What Units of Measurement" (2012), "What's a Byte" (2017), and the Dictionary of IBM and Computing Terminology (IBM, n.d.b.)

** A bit is either the digit "0" or the digit "1" (one binary unity) in the binary numeration system (IBM, n.d.b., p. 8); however, the values for coding may also be "no" and "yes" or some other binary options. A byte is "a string that consists of a number of bits, treated as a unit, and representing a character" (IBM, n.d.b., p. 10).

Corporations can use technology to capture unique and previously uncaptured data through technology that is currently in use: mobile devices, computers, Websites, medical equipment, and security hardware. Through technology, communication that was previously private—from sender to receiver—has moved into the public world of the Internet and allows users to interact anywhere on the planet. This interaction allows for diverse and numerous big data sources that include hardware *and* software. Mobile devices like phones track conversations, participants' identities and locations, and timing and length of interactions. "Those who use mobile technologies in the future will continue to build this record of themselves, creating outlines of lives and patterns of predictability" (Oppegaard, 2015, pp. 49–50). Other technologies—such as desktop and laptop computers and tablets—also track users' behaviors when the technologies are connected to the Internet; they record users' locations, searches, use of technologies, and buying and communicating practices through analytics (Davis, 2015). Other tools that gather data include

- biometrics—electronic devices that protect an individual's privacy (such as fingerprint, iris, and retina scanners and face recognition software; Singer, 2012);
- wearable devices that monitor a patient's physiologic and vital signs, such as an activity tracker that measures movement and heartrate, a continuous positive airway pressure (CPAP) machine that monitors an individual's sleep patterns and breathing at night, and a pacemaker transmitter that monitors a patient's heart activity;
- Websites and social media that gather data about individuals' online behavior.

Corporations are using big data—immense amounts of data gathered—to verify identity, to predict behavior, and to create better systems for the future.

Biometrics have been used since 2004 by the U.S. government for big data that Homeland Security uses. This data helps U.S. intelligence agencies to track questionable individuals and manage identities (U.S. Department of Homeland Security, 2009), but biometric tracking is also used in security systems and in financial institutions for security; that data is stored for documentation. Biometrics are also used on Facebook through face recognition so individuals can "tag" friends in their photographs—data that links networks of people through their Facebook profiles. Face-recognition software is also being proposed as a tool to help airlines improve their processes for checking in: JetBlue has tested face-recognition software to check passengers in (Yahoo View, 2017), and Delta Airlines is testing a "bio-metric-based baggage drop system" (Zhang, 2017). The data they collect will be stored to verify passengers' identity and perhaps to build a larger database of passenger records.

Wearable devices are being developed and improved quickly to improve medical care and to document trends with patients who use specific medical devices, such as CPAP machines, pacemakers, and neuromodulators. CPAP machines and pacemakers allow physicians to remotely monitor data about patients' physiologic performance; that data is also stored for documentation and analysis. This data is gathered, stored, and analyzed by appropriate parties who are given access to medical monitoring information.

And information gathered from websites and social media are typically publicly available or are available for sale. Big data can be sold to organizations that want to analyze the information per the organization's individual needs. Social media tools are free programs, but individuals do not use the tools without a cost. Every time a person uses technology, that individual submits to the agreement that the produced data is available for some level of data mining. The information may be protected, to be analyzed only by a particular organization that has permission to access the information. However, other information, publicly available information, may be analyzed or sold to other organizations that will analyze the data for the organization's benefit. Interactions and behaviors are not private unless individuals use tools that value privacy and allow users to use services without gathering information or who are legally required to protect the data.

Organizations and industries gather information by investing in the technology through which they collect data. They may provide free services, such as search engines or social networking, by providing the service or by advertising or funding the services. Then, individuals who use those services "pay" a price with their information, as stated above; if they use the service, they give consent for the organization to observe their behaviors and mine data related to their technology use. For example, if a person uses Google to search for information about diabetes, she is using Google's search engine at no charge and giving Google access to her search parameters. Google can then use that information to build a profile for users like her; in that way, Google can gather information from the way she uses her computer to search—and she may be on the Internet eight to ten hours a day for work, personal projects, communication, research, shopping, etc. Google creates technologies that she needs and then tracks her as she uses them. As individuals use the services, they begin to depend on the technology: for banking, communicating, shopping, driving, using a phone, etc. Every interaction via technology now creates data that is being captured.

A profile, or *persona*, can help an organization to create a picture that describes a potential audience member or client and thus helps the organization to design services, products, and marketing that is catered to that profiled audience. A profile includes demographic information that includes age, gender, ethnicity, socioeconomic level, education, and other "who" data; geographic or "where" data that matches online activity with an individual's location through Internet access point; and "what" and "how" behaviors that include an individual's purchase history and patterns as well as financial transactions. Profiles are necessary for organizations to focus on and expand their markets: to understand untouched markets, to improve communication with audiences, and to predict future trends.

By predicting future trends, corporations can create algorithms that predict what audiences want or suggest choices for potential services and products. For example, if an individual searches for nutrition information, then she might find advertisements for nutrition bars, dieting systems, and local gyms on her Facebook page. If she searches for books related to nutrition on Barnes & Noble or Amazon, she may find that the bookseller suggests other books related to those she chooses. Algorithms are steps embedded in computer code that instruct the Website of responses as a user makes a choice—to respond to the user's choices.

BIG DATA, HEALTH, AND MEDICINE

Big data related to medicine exists in government sites that can be accessed for no cost. For example, healthdata.gov provides "125 years of U.S. healthcare data including claim-level Medicare data, epidemiology, and population statistics," and the NHS Health and Social Care Information Centre provides data sets related to health in the United Kingdom (Marr, 2014). Other government sites provide health-related information. Organizations (such as health departments, pharmaceutical and medical supply companies, insurance companies, large physician pools, and medical-data management services) are also gathering health-related and medical information by mining data and analyzing and querying data to separate out health data or by gathering data from sites that focus on health information. This process, called *health analytics*, captures information related to pharmaceutical data, EMRs, and insurance and government-funding claims. Health analytics follow the same practices of data mining that other industries use, but they focus their analysis on costs, behaviors, and outcomes to focus on medical costs and trends and to establish customized medical experiences—"personalized medicine" that allows physicians to tailor treatment "to the individual characteristics of each patient. . . . Preventive and therapeutic interventions can then be concentrated on those who will benefit, sparing expense and side effects for those who will not" (Dulin, Hugh-Jones, Pitts, and Hughes, n.d., p. 2). Health data can be used to identify and predict health trends, to understand patients holistically, to assess treatment protocols, to provide return-on-investment to employers, to develop new models and products, and to improve care through "analytics-driven medical insights" (Dulin, Hugh-Jones, Pitts, and Hughes, n.d.). Analytics can also allow for healthcare institutions to evaluate workflow within the facility or to analyze outcomes to identify "standard-of-care issues" (Fornell, 2016). Analytics will also enable analysts to identify potential patients, even before those patients report symptoms, by identifying persona and then noting patients who fit into that persona (Fornell, 2016). In this way, big data can help to track patients and to anticipate disease patterns with great detail because analysis will be able to consider larger bodies of data (Butler, 2014).

These insights allow for expanded pharmaceutical and medical research that benefits patients through pointed product and care development, sales, and provision. In addition, data can help insurance companies to understand patient demand and company profitability and to predict future trends through statistics-supported predictions.

> Advanced data management and predictive analytics enable data-driven decisions that will allow health plans to adapt to new market realities by fully understanding the new dynamics and applying them to their unique portfolios of business—from predicting and managing shifts in the customer base, to transitioning from a wholesale to a consumer marketplace, to bending the cost curve through health and condition management, to detecting and preventing fraud, and beyond. (SAS Institute Inc., n.d.)

Analysis of medical data can also help us self-track our health and well-being through applications that allow us to track our own data (self-reported) or through sensors and gadgets that gather our personal data automatically to help us track our habits related to sleep and eating, sex, fertility, moods, and normal mechanisms like glucose and oxygen levels and blood pressure (Walker, 2015). In the United States, 60 percent of adults track diet, weight, and exercise, and 60 percent track their health; and in the United Kingdom, 70 percent track their health. In the United Kingdom, 25 percent of adults (25–44 years of age) reported that their health choices would be influenced by motivational prompts on their smartphones (Walker, 2015). Humans are creating and tracking data, and messages related to trends might encourage individuals to eat better, exercise more, and take care of themselves—behaviors that would improve their health. By analyzing medically focused data, analysts can work with healthcare policy makers, physicians, hospitals, insurance companies, and patients to improve care and resources and increase efficiency, thus decreasing costs. Per analyst justifications, big data benefits everyone in the medical system.

Big data related to medicine can help predict trends by organizing and comparing data related to side effects, diagnoses, medical histories, and other elements that otherwise would not be analyzed because the amount is too large for analysis. Recent research shows that analysis of big data predicted potential risks that are related to metabolic syndrome. By reviewing large amounts of data provided by a large insurance company, data scientists are identifying new risks, which allows the insurance company to develop and implement health programs that can alleviate those risks and thus decrease the incidence of this disease (Steinberg, Church, McCall, Scott, and Kalis, 2014). With analysis software that can identify previously missed correlations, these processes can help to identify medical trends that, if providers know, can help them to anticipate patterns of morbidity and even mortality and to develop preventive measures for their patients. The benefits are innumerable; insurance companies can find previously unidentified variables and correlations in data from large populations of patients and thus forecast risks that patients may face or illnesses that patients may experience. This enables preventive measures that can make the general population healthier and can improve preventive medicine. In fact, Google analysts predict that the United States decreased its patient mortality from flu by 20 percent by analyzing live-streamed data on patients being diagnosed with the flu (Walker, 2015).

Epidemiologists and data scientists are already starting to experiment with big data to analyze information and identify health-related issues. As early as 2008, a group of researchers and physicians from the University of Minnesota and a partnering practice ran a simulation of software to predict treatment errors related to encounters and care related to patients with type 2 diabetes. Using already existing patient records, the researchers created a synthetic population of ten thousand patients and then applied physician process models to identify which were the most and least effective. In this study,

> specific data mining model (a decision tree) was developed to predict errors of omission that occurred throughout the patient population by virtue of different treatment strategies. . . . The ability to interpret how an error is predicted has implications for the formation of policies based on these predictions.
> An important aspect of the work presented here is the fact that physician and patient models were used to generate simulated encounter data from which data mining tools could be developed. . . . have the potential to enable identification and correction of physician decision-making strategies that lead to encounter-specific treatment errors. (McCabe, Adomavicius, Johnson, et al., 2008, p. 15)

The researchers report that they pilot the data-mining prediction tool on a database of 77,514 patient records from 12,708 real-life patients treated by 129 physicians. After refining the data set to usable data and running the tool, with a recall of errors to be 67 percent (compared to 61 percent in the synthetic study). Although this tool does not offer a refined method for analyzing large amounts of data, it does improve the analytics for evidence-based assessment of patient and physician encounters.

In 2015, Kaur and Bawa published findings of a study to identify data-mining methods and tools and to answer question about the future trends of data mining. The investigators report a list of data-mining tools used in medical studies: Weka, Tanagra, Orange, R, Rapid Miner, and Knime (p. 21). The tools exist, and researchers are already using them in studies (as early as 2005) to investigate trends related to cancer (breast, skin, and lung); heart disease; diabetes; hepatitis; dialysis; and liver disorders (Kaur and Bawa, 2015, p. 23) and to report prediction accuracies between 52 percent and 94 percent (Kaur and Bawa, 2015, pp. 24–26). Their study reports accuracy with medical records in a major constraint in accurate data analysis; therefore, errors and outliers do influence results when analyzing large amounts of data. However, perhaps most telling from this study is the growing trend for data analysis as it relates to medical data and the potential benefits that big data can bring to the medical community.

BIG DATA AND PATIENTHOOD

Not all outcomes from big data are positive. Patients complicate the control of their personal information when they disclose protected information online. Participating in medically focused, and particularly diagnosis-specific, online communities, individuals seek to fit into the community and thus share information to qualify as a valid member of the patient group. They may share information that would be protected if transferred by medical institutions, practitioners, or insurance providers; however, patients have the freedom to own their medical information and they can self-disclose that information as they choose.

As patients in online communities share information, the members of the audience become co-owners of the shared information. The audience can be the intended recipient of the information—perhaps an individual or a small group of discoursing patients who are sharing information. (I see this in the threads I analyze on Breastcancer.org, as women share information with the other members of the online community in an effort to ask questions, share experience, create community, and develop relationships.) Intended audiences most likely respect information and thus protect it, not gathering information solely for their own benefit or to do harm to the sender; they consider the relational value of the message and, because of the rhetorical elements of the community—members seeking to fit in by building their *logos*, *ethos*, and *pathos*—they value the community and their place within the community.

Unintended audiences, however, have no such loyalty or relational motivation: they do not invest in the other members by interacting, and they do not participate in the discourse. They exist in the online space to observe and gather information, with no accountability for the way they use the information that they gather. They do not need to establish their credibility, logically work through community-shared concerns and issues, or share the emotional elements of the focus of the community. Unintended audiences are a particular concern when they have access to information from a public (non-password-protected) community because they have open access to any information shared; they do not log into the space or leave a trace when they visit and have no responsibility to the community through relationship. Public communities are open to anyone with Internet access. Anyone can visit the community, observe the text-based discourse in that space, and leave with information. In public forums for superficial or non-sensitive information—such as product feedback, game-centric conversations, movie reviews, and comments about news and food—the open access is less of an issue; however, in a medically focused or diagnosis-specific community where individuals experiencing patienthood are sharing private information, the open access can be a thread to patients' security, confidentiality, and privacy. Patients, not considering the "unseen" and unintended audiences, may disclose information that they would otherwise not publicly share.

As data is mined from the Internet and as medical data is siphoned from big data, individuals who share their experiences in these public communities are caught up as subjects of this data, and their illness narratives are gathered by unintended audiences. Their illness narratives become raw data: to be coded, analyzed, clustered, and categorized. As raw data, the ownership of the patients' illness narratives is now passed to an unintended audience for unintended purposes that might potentially harm the members of the community. Their medical history, what is now pre-existing data, can become a liability if the illness narrative and related information can be traced back to the individual.

This disclosure is disconcerting, as noted in chapter 4, because community members create privacy risks for themselves; identifiable information merged with identifiers allow anyone to create profiles of individuals in the community. Some members may think this is paranoia: "Who would waste time gathering information about me?" But data and information equal power, and corporations that gather valuable information increase their value and their ability to sell and trade information. Additionally, if data scientists are encouraged to "swim" through data for unique findings, they may find some of the most personal and specific data in publicly published illness narratives.

Patienthood is not changing; humans will still face illness and need to depend on trained physicians to provide the healthcare that they need to overcome illnesses. Online communities are changing—they are growing. As the medical field chooses to move away from a paternalistic model to one of partnership with the patient and to a business model that considers the patient as a client and patient satisfaction to be a primary goal, patients will be required to investigate more to participate. Thus, patienthood on the Internet will expand as individuals who are seeking medical information in a language they can understand learn more about their diagnoses and about what they can expect in the disease processes. In addition, disease narratives will be investigated as therapeutic possibilities and physicians, particularly practitioners encouraging more naturalistic therapies, will encourage patients to share their stories; the Internet is a natural place for patients to share their stories because they can interact in structured environments with others who are empathetic per their stories.

Individuals online believe their information is private; they do not acknowledge that their online content can be accessed, mined, and shared (Butler, McCann, and Thomas, n.d.; Cate, 2010; Gelman, 2009; Goldsborough, 2010; Ji and Lieber, 2010; Kamakshi and Babu, 2010; Levin and Abril, 2009; McCullagh, 2009; Mohamed, 2010; Sundar and Marathe, 2010; Whitehouse, 2010). They are spending more time online, as work requires and growing leisure time allows; they are spending more time online (Walmsley, 2000). Perhaps leisure time and the amount of time individuals are conducting work on the Internet expands the size of the Internet. Therefore, as individuals continue to seek information on the Internet and as it continues to grow, the body of medical information will also expand.

As the Internet expands, online research will expand. Researchers will gather more information to learn how individuals in online spaces behave (Segal, 2005). Research methods will continue to need expansion, from standard protocols for social science research to adapted methods that allow for Internet research. At the same time, standardizing bodies such as IRBs will need to adapt their protocols for approval to allow for online artifacts to be accepted and to consider the ethical dilemmas that are unique to online texts. As research expands and as the Internet and its participant pool expands, big data will expand. More corporations will design software to mine and analyze data and hardware to store large amounts of data. Thus, more information will be released to unintended audiences.

Privacy will become an issue on the Internet; anything posted will be replicable, and individuals cannot expect their comments and stories to be protected if they post the sensitive information themselves. Some communities will respond and, although they will be limiting access, they will create security systems, such as password-protected areas; this will decrease the sites' ability to draw search engines, and it will also decrease their liability in regards to the security of information that their community members post.

If physicians want to increase their knowledge of patient feedback, they will begin to consider what patients are saying in their own "backstage" as they interact in online communities. The information will help physicians better understand how patients respond to different approaches to medicine, and they can then adapt their bedside manner to meet patients demands and expectations. However, in mining information about patient responses, physicians will also make that information more readily available to insurance and pharmaceutical companies, a continuance of the security issues that are so dangerous to patients today. The response may be for patients to stop sharing their narratives in open-access communities. There is no way to know how patients will respond.

Patienthood needs to be something that individuals share but guardedly. They need to share their illness narratives—benefiting themselves and helping others who struggle with their own experiences—and yet guard personal information that can compromise their privacy. Members of medically focused online communities need to decrease the personal and identifiable information that they share, ensuring that they use pseudonyms that do not lead others to their true identities. They need to know and to remember that unintended audiences are constantly taking co-ownership of the information that they share and, as a result, they should decrease information about their geographic locations, their families, their medical histories, and other personal information that help to build their *ethos* and *pathos* within the community but that can also be a liability in their security and privacy. They can simplify the information they share about their current diagnosis, their medical history, their disease process, and their personal lives, saving disclosure for discourse behind passwords and in secure spaces—so they can control their information. Members in online communities can do this—if they integrate considerations of privacy into the rhetoric of breast cancer.

NOTE

1. The job of data scientist is considered "the sexiest job of the 21st century" (Davenport and Patil, 2012). Data scientists recognize that they will face technology limitations and need to think creatively to overcome obstacles and enjoy "swimming" through large amounts of data to explore and learn (Davenport and Patil, 2012).

References

About Breastcancer.org: History, leadership, site features. (2016, January 27). *Breastcancer.org*. Retrieved from http://www.Breastcancer.org/about_us/press_room/press_kit/about_bco.jsp.

Active. (2010, October 29). RE: I belong to an online community at monome.org [Online forum content]. Retrieved from http://post.monome.org/comments.php?DiscussionID=9664.

Adesina, A. O., Agbele, K. K., Februarie, R., Abidoye, A. P., and Nyongesa, H. O. (2011). Ensuring the security and privacy of information in mobile health-care communication systems. *South African Journal of Science, 107*(9/10), 1–7.

Agency. (n.d.). *Dictionary and thesaurus—Merriam-Webster online*. Retrieved from http://www.merriam-webster.com/dictionary/agency.

Alkureishi, M. A., Lee, W. W., Lyons, M., Press, V. G., Iman, S., Nkansah-Amankra, A., Werner, D., and Arora, V. M. (2016). Impact of electronic medical record use on the patient–doctor relationship and communication: A systematic review. *Journal of General Internal Medicine, 31*(5), 548–60. doi: 10.1007/211606-015-03582-1.

American Cancer Society, Inc. (2016). *Cancer information on the Internet.* Retrieved from http://www.cancer.org/cancer/cancerbasics/cancer-information-on-the-internet.

Anderson, A. S., and Klemm, P. (2008). The Internet: Friend or foe when providing patient education? *Clinical Journal of Oncology Nursing, 12*(1), 55–63.

Angeli, E. L. (2012). Metaphors in the rhetoric of pandemic flu: Electronic media coverage of H1N1 and swine flu. *Journal of Technical Writing and Communication, 42*(3), 203–22. doi: 10.2190/TW.42.3.b.

Angeli, E., and Johnson-Sheehan, R. (2017). CFP for special issue of TCQ. *Rhetoricians of Health and Medicine HomePage.* Retrieved from http://medicalrhetoric.com/cfp-for-special-issue-of-tcq.

Antaki, C., Barnes, R., and Leudar, I. (2005). Self-disclosure as a situated interactional practice. *British Journal of Social Psychology, 44,* 181–99.

Antiphon. (2010, October 29). RE: I belong to an online community at monome.org [Online forum content]. Retrieved from http://post.monome.org/comments.php?DiscussionID=9664.

Anton, A. I., Breaux, T. D., Gritzalis, S., and Mylopoulos, J. (2011). Digital privacy, Theory, policies and technologies. *Requirements Engineering, 16,* 1–2. doi: 10.1007/s00766-011-0117-0.

Anwar, F., Chae, H. S., and Natriello, G. (2010). NetPosse: A tool for connecting users in virtual communities. *Systemics, Cybernetics and Informatics, 8*(1), 67–71.B

Arduser, L. (2011). Warp and Weft: Weaving the Discussion Threads of an Online Community. *Journal of Technical Writing and Communication, 41*(1), 5–31.

Arduser, L. (2017). *Living chronic: Agency and expertise in the rhetoric of diabetes*. Columbus, OH: The Ohio State University Press.

Aristotle. (n.d.). *Nichomachean Ethics* (W. D. Ross, Trans.). New York: Modern Library. (Original work published 350 BCE) Retrieved from http://classics.mit.edu/Aristotle/nicomachaen.html.

Aristotle. (1924). *Rhetoric* (W. R. Roberts, Trans.). New York, NY: Modern Library. (Original work published 350 BCE). Retrieved from http://classics.mit.edu/Aristotle/rhetoric.3.iii.html.

Aristotle. (2004). *The art of rhetoric* (H. C. Lawson-Tancred, Trans.). London, England: Penguin Books. (Original work published 350 BCE).

Ashing-Giwa, K. T., and Lim, J.-W. (2010). Exploring the association between functional strain and emotional well-being among a population-based sample of breast cancer survivors. *Psycho-Oncology, 19,* 150–59. doi: 10.1002/pon.1517.

Attrill, A., and Jalil, R. (2011). Revealing only the superficial me: Exploring categorical self-disclosure online. *Computers in Human Behavior, 27,* 1634–42.

Bakardjieva, M. (2007). Virtual togetherness: An everyday-life perspective. In D. Bell and B. M. Kennedy (Eds.), *The cybercultures reader* (2nd ed.) (pp. 236–53). London, UK: Routledge.

Ballard-Reisch, D. S., and Letner, J. A. (2003). Centering families in cancer communication research: Acknowledging the impact of support, culture and process on client/provider communication in cancer management. *Patient Education and Counseling, 50,* 61–66.

Bandi, P., Brinton, L., Buchert, S., Cokkinides, V., Cowens-Alavarado, R., Elk, R., et al. (2009). *Breast cancer facts & figures: 2009–2010.* Atlanta, GA: American Cancer Society, Inc.

Bartle, P. (2007). What is community? A sociological perspective. *Seattle Community Network.* Retrieved from http://www.scn.org/cmp/whatcom.htm.

Barton, E. (2001). Design in observational research on the discourse of medicine: Toward disciplined interdisciplinarity. *Journal of Business and Technical Communication, 15,* 309–32.

Barton, E. (2004). Discourse methods and critical practice in professional communication: The front-stage and back-stage discourse of prognosis in medicine. *Journal of Business and Technical Communication, 18,* 67–111. doi: 101177/1050651903258127.

Barton, E. (2005). Introduction to the special issue: The discourses of medicine. *Journal of Business and Technical Communication, 19*(3), 245–48. doi: 10.1177/1050651905275636.

Barton, E. (2007). Disability narratives of the law: Narratives and counter-narratives. *Narrative, 15*(1), 95–112.

Bazeley, P. (2007). *Qualitative data analysis with NVivo.* Thousand Oaks, CA: Sage Publications, Inc.

Beaudoin, C. E., and Tao, C.-C. (2007). Benefiting from social capital in online support groups: An empirical study of cancer patients. *CyberPsychology & Behavior, 10,* 587–90.

Beddows, E. (2008). The methodological issues associated with Internet-based research. *International Journal of Emerging Technologies and Society, 6*(2), 124–39.

Bell, D. (2001). *An introduction to cybercultures.* New York: Routledge.

Bellwoar, H. (2012). Everyday Matters: Reception and Use as Productive Design of Health-Related Texts. *Technical Communication Quarterly, 21,* 325–45.

Ben-Arye, E., Traube, Z., Schachter, L., Motti, H., Levy, M., Schiff, E., and Lev, E. (2011). Integrative pediatric care: Parents' attitudes toward communication of physicians and CAM practitioners. *Pediatrics, 127,* e84–e95. doi: 10.1542/eds.2010-1286.

Berle, I. (2011). Privacy and confidentiality: What is the difference? *Journal of Visual Communication in Medicine, 34,* 43–44. doi: 10.3109/17453054.2011.550845.

Bernard, D. S., Farr, S. L., and Fang, Z. (2011). National estimates of out-of-pocket health care expenditure burdens among nonelderly adults with cancer: 2001 to 2008. *Journal of Clinical Oncology.* doi: 10.1200/jco.2010.33.0522.

Bertakis, K. D. (2009). The influence of gender on the doctor–patient interaction. *Patient Education Counseling, 76*, 356–60.

Biermann, J. S., Golladay, G. J., Greenfield, M. L. V. H., and Baker, L. H. (1999). Evaluation of cancer information on the Internet. *Cancer, 86*, 381–90.

Birnhack, M., and Elkin-Koren, N. (2011, May 25). Does law matter online? Empirical evidence on privacy law compliance. *Michigan Telecommunications and Technology Law Review, 17*, 337–84. Retrieved from http://www.mttlr.org/volseventeen/birnhack&elkin-koren.pdf.

Blakeslee, A. M., and Spilka, R. (2004). The state of research in technical communication. *Technical Communication Quarterly, 13*, 73–92.

Blank, T. O., and Adams-Blodnieks, M. (2007). The who and the what of usage of two cancer online communities. *Computers in Human Behavior, 23*, 1249–57.

Blobel, B. (2011). Intelligent security and privacy solutions for enabling personalized telepathology. *Diagnostic Pathology, 6*(suppl), 1–8. Retrieved from http://www.diagnosticpathology.org/content/6/S1/S4.

Bodle, R. (2011). Privacy and participation in the cloud: Ethical implications of Google's privacy practices and public communications. In B. E. Drushel and K. German (Eds.), The ethics of emerging media: Information, social norms, and new media technology (pp. 155–74). New York: The Continuum International Publishing Group.

Bhoo-Pathy, N., Harman, M., Yip, C.-H., Saxena, N., Taib, N. A., Lim, S.-E., et al. (2012). Ethnic differences in survival after breast cancer in South East Asia. *PLoS ONE 7*(2), e3099f. doi: 10.1371/journal.pone.0030995.

Borzekowski, D. L. G., Schenk, S., Wilson, J. L., and Peebles, R. (2010). e-Ana and e-Mia: A content analysis of pro-eating disorder Web sites. *American Journal of Public Health, 100*(8), 1526–34.

Bowman-Grieve, L. (2009). Exploring "Stormfront": A virtual community of the radical right. *Studies in Conflict & Terrorism, 32*, 989–1007. doi: 10.1080/1057610090329951.

Boyles, S. (2007, October 22). Positive attitude doesn't whip cancer? [Web log]. *WebMD.* Retrieved from http://www.webmd.com/cancer/news/20071022/positive-attitude-doesnt-whip-cancer#1.

Bradley, C. J., Dahman, B., Shickle, L. M., and Lee, W. (2012). Surgery wait times and specialty services for insured and uninsured breast cancer patients: Does hospital safety net status matter? *HSR: Health Services Research, 47*, 677–97. doi: 10.1111/j.1475-6773.2011.01328.x.

Bradley, S. M. (2008). The Internet: Can patients link to credible resources? *MEDSURG Nursing, 17*(4), 229–36.

Breastcancer.org. (2011). *Aromatase inhibitors.* Retrieved from http://www.Breastcancer.org/treatment/hormonal/aromatase_inhibitors/index.jsp.

Breastcancer.org. (2017). *Wigs.* Retrieved from http://www.breastcancer.org/tips/hair_skin_nails/wigs.

Breastcancer.org Community. (2016, October 31). *Community.* Retrieved from http://www.Breastcancer.org/community.

Breastcancer.org—Community Guidelines. (2016). *Rules*. Retrieved from https://community.breastcancer.org/help/rules.

Breastcancer.org Team. (2016). *About us—Team.* Retrieved from http://www.breastcancer.org/about_us/team.

Bump. (2011a). *BreastFeeding.com community.* Retrieved from http://www.breastfeeding.com/community.aspx.

Bump. (2011b). *BreastFeeding.com terms & conditions* Retrieved from http://www.breastfeeding.com/social/popup/file_terms/dir_language.

Bunde, M., Suis, J., Martin, R., and Barnett, K. (2006). Hystersisters online: Social support and social comparison among hysterectomy patients on the Internet. *Annals of Behavioral Medicine, 31*(3), 271–78. doi: 10.1207/s15324796abm3103_9.

Burke, K. (1969). The rhetoric of motives. Sacramento, CA: University of California Press.

Butler, E., McCann, E., and Thomas, J. (n.d.). Privacy setting awareness on Facebook and its effect on user-posted content. *Human Communication, 14*(1), 39–55.

Butler, M. (2014, November 1). HIM's Role in Disease Tracking, Data Mining, and Patient Monitoring. *AHIMA*. Retrieved from http://journal.ahima.org/2014/11/01/hims-role-in-disease-tracking-data-mining-and-patient-monitoring.

Bury, M. (2001). Illness narratives: Fact or fiction? *Sociology of Health & Illness, 23*(3), 263–85. doi: 10.1111/1467-9566.00252.

Byrn, T. (2008). Thinking out of the box about communities. *EContentMag*. 60. Retrieved from http://www.econtentmag.com/Articles/ArticleReader.aspx?ArticleID=51625.

Cahill, R. (2008, March). Survey: Online breast cancer information not always accurate. *Distinctions.* Retrieved from http://www.uthouston.edu/distinctions/archive/2008/march/archive.htm?id=591326.

Campbell, K. K. (2005). Agency: Promiscuous and protean. *Communication and Critical/Cultural Studies, 2,* 3.

Cancerhelp UK. (2010). *FEC.* Retrieved from http://cancerhelp.cancerresearchuk.org/about-cancer/treatment/cancer-drugs/fec_.

Cancernet–uk. (n.d.). *AC-Taxol.* Retrieved from http://www.cancernet.co.uk/chem-ac-taxol.htm.

Carlat, D. (2013). Hot topics in pharmaceutical industry ethics. Psych Central . Retrieved from https://pro.psychcentral.com/hot-topics-in-pharmaceutical-industry-ethics/004479.html.

Carter, D. (2005). Living in virtual communities: An ethnography of human relationships in cyberspace. *Information, Communication & Society, 8,* 148–67. doi: 10.1080/13691180500146235.

Carter, D. M. (2004). Living in virtual communities: Making friends online. *Journal of Urban Technology, 11*(3), 109–25. doi: 10.1080/10630730500064448.

Cassidy, L. (2011). Online communities of practice to support collaborative mental health practice in rural areas. *Issues in Mental Health Nursing, 32,* 98–107. doi: 10.33109/01612840.2010.535648.

Cate, F. H. (2010). Protecting privacy in health research: The limits of individual choice. *California Law Review, 98,* 1765–1803.

Charles, C., Gafni, A., and Whelan, T. (2000). How to improve communication between doctors and patients: Learning more about the decision making context is important. *British Medical Journal, 320,* 1220–21.

Chen, G. M. (2012). Why do women write personal blogs? Satisfying needs for self-disclosure and affiliation tell part of the story. *Computers in Human Behavior, 28,* 171–80.

Child, J. T., Pearson, J. C., and Petrionio, S. (2009). Blogging, communication, and privacy management: Development of the blogging privacy management measure. *Journal of the American Society for Information Science and Technology, 60,* 2079–94.

Chou, S.-W., Min, H.-T., Chang, Y.-C., and Lin, C.-T. (2010). Understanding continuance intention of knowledge creation using extended expectation–confirmation theory: An empirical study of Taiwan and China online communities. *Behaviour & Information Technology, 29,* 557–70. doi: 10.1080/01449290903401986.

Chouchane, L., Boussen, H., and Sastry, K. S. R. (2013). Breast cancer in Arab populations: Molecular characteristics and disease management implications. *Lancet Oncology, 14,* e417–e424.

Clark, S. (1994). *Japan, a view from the bath.* Honolulu, HI: University of Hawaii Press. Retrieved from http://muse.jhu.edu/book/7939.

Cline, R. J. W., and Haynes, K. M. (2001). Consumer health information seeking on the Internet: The state of the art. *Health Education Research, 16*(6), 671–92.

Coe, C. (1998). Defending community: Difference and Utopia online. *International Journal of Cultural Studies, 1,* 391–414. doi: 10.1177/136787799800100305.

Community. (2012). *Dictionary and thesaurus—Merriam-Webster online*. Retrieved from http://www.merriam-webster.com/dictionary/community.

Compelling. (n.d.) *Dictionary.com*. Retrieved from http://www.dictionary.com/browse/compelling.

CostHelper, Inc. (2017a). *Breast cancer treatment cost.* Retrieved from http://health.costhelper.com/breast-cancer.html.

CostHelper, Inc. (2017b). *How much does breast reconstruction cost?* Retrieved from http://health.costhelper.com/breast-reconstruction.html.

Costigan, J. T. (1999). Introduction: Forests, trees, and Internet research. In Jones, S. (Ed.), *Doing Internet research: Critical issues and methods for examining the net* (pp. xvii–xxiv). Thousand Oaks, CA: SAGE Publications.

Coughlin, S. S., and Ekwueme, D. U. (2009). Breast cancer as a global health concern. *Cancer Epidemiology, 33*, 315–18. doi: 10.1016/j.canep.2009.10.003

Cousin, G., Mast, M. S., Roter, D. L., and Hall, J. A. (2012). Concordance between physician communication style and patient attitudes predicts patient satisfaction. *Patient Education Counseling, 87*, 193–97.

Creswell, J. W. (2009). *Research design: Qualitative, quantitative, and mixed methods approaches* (3rd ed.). Thousand Oaks, CA: Sage Publications, Inc.

Dalton and Dalton. (1975). *Community and its relevance to Australian society*. Canberra, Australia: Australian Government Publishing Service.

Davenport, T. H., and Patil, D. J. (2012). Data scientist: The sexiest job of the 21st century. *Harvard Business Review*. Retrieved from https://hbr.org/2012/10/data-scientist-the-sexiest-job-of-the-21st-century.

Davis, J. (2015). Marketing, communication, and corporate media. In C. S. Lambert and M. Schlobohm, *Communication and emerging media: What's trending now*. Dubuque, IA: Kendall Hunt Publishers.

Debatin, B., Lovejoy, J. P., Horn, A.-K., and Hughes, B. N. (2009). Facebook and online privacy: Attitudes, behaviors, and unintended consequences. *Journal of Computer-Mediated Communication, 15*, 83–108. doi: 10.1111/j.1083.2009.01494.x.

de Jong, M. D. T. (2009). Practically meaningful academic research and academically relevant practitioner research. *Technical Communication, 56*(2), 97–98.

de Kok, M., Dirksen, C. D., Kessels, A. G., van der Weijden, T., van de Velde, C. J., Roukema, J. A., Bell, A. V., van der Ent, F. W., and von Meyenfeldt, M. F. (2010). Cost-effectiveness of a short stay admission programme for breast cancer surgery. *Acta Oncologica, 49*, 338–46. doi: 10.3109/02841861003610192.

Delanty, G. (2010). *Community*. New York: Taylor & Francis.

Derkatch, C. (2012). Demarcating medicine's boundaries: Constituting and categorizing in the journals of the American Medical Association. *Technical Communication Quarterly, 21*, 210–29.

Derkatch, C. (2015). Bounding biomedicine: Evidence and rhetoric in the new science of alternative medicine. Chicago, IL: University of Chicago Press.

Derkatch, C., and Segal, J. Z. (2005). Realms of rhetoric in health and medicine. *University of Toronto Medical Journal, 82*(2), 138–42.

Deshields, T., Rihanek, A., Potter, P., Zhang, Q., Kuhrik, M., Kuhrik, N., and O'Neill, J. (2012). Psychosocial aspects of caregiving: Perceptions of cancer patients and family caregivers. *Support Care Center, 20*, 349–56. doi: 10.1007/s00520-01101092-1.

DHHS. (2003, May). OCR privacy brief: Summary of the HIPAA Privacy Rule. Washington, D.C.: U.S. Department of Health and Human Services. Retrieved from http://www.hhs.gov/ocr/privacy/hipaa/understanding/summary/index.html/privacysummary.pdf.

Dickerson, S. S., Alquaissi, N., Underhill, M., and Lally, R. M. (2011). Surviving the wait: Defining support while awaiting breast cancer surgery. *Journal of Advanced Nursing, 67*, 1468–79. doi: 10.1111/j.1365-2648.2011.05612.x.

Dickerson, S. S., Boehmke, M., Ogle, C., Brown, J. K. (2006). Seeking and managing hope: Patients' experiences using the Internet for cancer care. *Oncology Nursing Forum, 33*(1), E8–E17.

Dibbell, J. (n.d.). *A rape in cyberspace: How an evil clown, a Haitian trickster spirit, two wizards, and a cast of dozens turned a database into a society*. Retrieved from http://www.juliandibbell.com/texts/bungle_vv.html.

Dickerson, S. S., Boehmke, M., Ogle, C., and Brown, J. K. (2006). Seeking and managing hope: Patients' experiences using the Internet for cancer care. *Oncology Nursing Forum, 33*(1), E8–E17.

Ding, H. (2009). Rhetorics of alternative media in an emerging epidemic: SARS, censorship, and extra-institutional risk communication. *Technical Communication Quarterly, 18,* 327–50.

Dinolfo, J., Heifferon, B., and Temesvari, L. A. (2007). Seeing cells: Teaching the visual/verbal rhetoric of biology. *Journal of Technical Writing and Communication, 37*(4), 395–417.

Discourse. (n.d.). *Etymonline.com.* Retrieved from http://www.etymonline.com/index.php?term=discourse.

Donne, J. (1999). "Devotions upon emergent occasions" and "Death's duel" with "The life of Dr. John Donne" by Izaak Walton. New York: Random House.

Dulin, M., Hugh-Jones, C., Pitts, M., and Hughes, G. (n.d.). *Applying data to improve patient-centric and personalized medicine: Conclusions paper.* Retrieved from https://www.sas.com/content/dam/SAS/en_us/doc/conclusionpaper1/applying-data-improve-patient-centric-personalized-medicine-106556.pdf.

Dumont, G., and Candler, G. (2005). Virtual jungles: Survival, accountability, and governance in online communities. *The American Review of Public Administration, 35,* 287–99. doi: 10.1177.0275074005276350.

Durian, D. (2002). Corpus-based test analysis from a qualitative perspective: A closer look at NVivo. *Style, 36,* 738–42.

Eastin, M. S. (2001). Credibility assessments of online health information: The effects of source expertise and knowledge of content. *Journal of Computer-Mediated Communication, 6.* Retrieved from http://jcmc.indiana.edu/vol6/issue4/eastin.html.

Ebeling, M. F. E. (2003). The new dawn: Black agency in cyberspace. *Radical History Review, 87,* 96–108.

Egerod, I., Christensen, D., Schwartz-Nielsen, K., and Agard, A. (2011). Constructing the illness narrative: A grounded theory exploring patients' and relatives' use of intensive care diaries. *Critical Care Medicine, 39*(8), 1922–28. doi: 10.1097/CCM.0b013e31821e89c8.

Elm, M. S. (2009). "Question three: How do various notions of privacy influence decisions in qualitative Internet research?" In A. N. Markham and N. K. Baym (Eds.), *Internet inquiry: Conversations about method* (pp. 69–87). Thousand Oaks, CA: Sage Publications.

Farkas, K., and Haas, C. (2012). A grounded theory approach for studying writing and literacy. In K. Powell and P. Takayoshi (Eds.), *Practicing research in writing studies: Reflexive and ethically responsible research.* New York: Hampton Press.

Federal Bureau of Investigation. (n.d.). *What we investigate: Cyber crime.* Retrieved from https://www.fbi.gov/investigate/cyber.

Federal Trade Commission. (1998). *Children's Online Privacy Protection Act of 1998, 15 U.S.C. 6501–6505.* Retrieved from https://www.ftc.gov/enforcement/rules/rulemaking-regulatory-reform-proceedings/childrens-online-privacy-protection-rule.

Fernbeck, J. (1999). There is a there there: Notes toward a definition of cybercommunity. In S. Jones (Ed.), *Doing Internet research: Critical issues and methods for examining the Net* (pp. 203–18). Thousand Oaks, CA: SAGE Publications, Inc.

Finfgeld, D. L. (2000). Therapeutic groups online: The good, the bad, and the unknown. *Issues in Mental Health Nursing, 21,* 241–55.

Fischer, K., and Yasin, K. (2016, November 11). Breast cancer by the numbers: Survival rates by stage, age, and country [Web log]. *HealthLine.* Retrieved from http://www.healthline.com/health/breast-cancer/survival-facts-statistics#1.

Fornell, D. (2016, April 10). Understanding how big data will change healthcare. *DAIC.* Retrieved from https://www.dicardiology.com/article/understanding-how-big-data-will-change-healthcare.

Fox, S., and Duggan, M. (2013). Health online 2013. *Pew Research Center: Internet & Technology.* Retrieved from http://www.pewinternet.org/2013/01/15/health-online-2013.

Gallagher, E. J. (2009, January 7). Shaping a culture of conversation: The discussion board and beyond. *Academic Commons.* Retrieved from http://www.academiccommons.org/commons/essay/shaping-culture-conversation.

Gammon, K. S. (2007, October 16). Women struggle with breast cancer expenses. *ABC-News.com*. Retrieved from http://abcnews.go.com/Health/OnCallPlus/story?id=3736060&page=1#.T0mWfMwZDV0.

Gangadharbatla, H. (2008). *Facebook* me: Collective self-esteem, need to belong, and Internet self-efficacy as predictors of the iGeneration's attitudes toward social networking sites. *Journal of Interactive Advertising, 8*(2). Retrieved from http://jiad.org/article100.

Garcia, A. C., Standlee, A. I., Bechkoff, J., and Cui, Y. (2009). Ethnographic approaches to the Internet and computer-mediated communication. *Journal of Contemporary Ethnography, 38*(1), 52–84. doi: 10.1177/0891241607310839.

Garden, R. (2010). Telling stories about illness and disability: The limits and lessons of narrative. Perspectives in Biology and Medicine, 53(1), 121–35. DOI: 10.1353/pbm.0.0135.

Garton, L., Haythornthwaite, C., and Wellman, B. (1997). Studying online social networks. *Journal of Computer-Mediated Communication, 3*. Retrieved from http://jcmc.indiana.edu/vol3/issue1/garton.html.

Garver, E. (2009). Aristotle on the kinds of rhetoric. *Rhetorica: A Journal of the History of Rhetoric, 27*(1), 1–18. doi: 10.1525/rh.2009.27.1.1.

Gáspárik, A. I., Ábrám, Z., Geana, D., Sebesi, S., Farcas, D., and Gáspárik, A. C. (2014). Shortages of doctor-patient communication: Teaching patients to communicate effectively. *Procedia—Social and Behavioral Sciences, 142*, 376–79. doi: 10.1016/j.sbspro.2014.07.693.

Gelman, L. (2009). Privacy, free speech, and "blurry-edged" social networks. *Boston College Law Review, 50*, 1315–44.

Giddens, A. (1984). The constitution of society: Outline of the theory of structuration. Berkeley, CA: University of California Press.

Gill, E. A., and Babrow, A. S. (2007). To hope or to know: Coping with uncertainty and ambivalence in women's magazine breast cancer articles. *Journal of Applied Communication Research, 35*, 133–55. doi: 10.1080/00909880701263029.

Given, B. A., Given, C. W., and Kozachik, S. (2001). Family support in advanced cancer. *Cancer Journal for Clinicians, 51*, 213–31.

Glaser, B. G., and Strauss, A. L. (2008). *The discovery of grounded theory: Strategies for qualitative research.* New Brunswick, NJ: Aldine Transaction.

Goldsborough, R. (2010). Are you protecting your privacy online? *Teacher Librarian, 37*, 72.

Goodsell, T. L., and Williams, O. (2008). The case of the Brick Huggers: The practice of an online community. *City & Community, 7*, 251–71.

Gorey, K. M., Luginaah, I. N., Holowaty, E. J., Fung, K. Y., and Hamm, C. (2009). Wait times for surgical and adjuvant radiation treatment of breast cancer in Canada and the United States: Greater socioeconomic inequity in America. *Clinical Investigative Medicine, 32*(3), E239–E249.

Goubil-Gambrell, P. (1992). A practitioner's guide to research methods. *Technical Communication, 4*, 582–91.

Graham, S. S. (2009). Agency and the rhetoric of medicine: Biomedical brain scans and the ontology of Fibromyalgia. *Technical Communication Quarterly, 18*, 376–404.

Gremore, T. M., Baucom, D. H., Porter, L. S., Kirby, J. S., Atkins, D. C., and Keefe, F. J. (2011). Stress buffering effects of daily spousal support on women's daily emotional and physical experiences in the context of breast cancer concerns. *Health Psychology, 30*(1), 20–30. doi: 10.1037/10021798.

Haas, C. (Ed). (2009). Special issue on writing and medicine. *Written Communication, 26*, 115–211.

Hader, A. L., and Brown, E. D. (2010). Patient privacy and social media. *American Association of Nurse Anesthetists Journal, 78*(4), 270–74.

Halstead, W. S. (1894). The results of operations for the cure of cancer of the breast performed at the Johns Hopkins Hospital from June, 1889, to January, 1894. *Annals of Surgery, 20*(5), 497–555. Retrieved from https://www.ncbi.nlm.nih.gov/pmc/articles/PMC1493925/pdf/annsurg01118-0002.pdf.

Hamman, R. (1997). Introduction to virtual communities research and *Cybersociology Magazine,* issue two. *Cybersociology Magazine, 2*. Retrieved from http://www.cybersociology.com/files/2_1_hamman.html.
Harper, D. (2016). Community. *Oxford etymology dictionary.* Retrieved from http://www.etymonline.com/index.php?term=community.
Harris, J. (2009, September 10). Experts debate if the cost of end-of-life cancer care is too high. *HemOnc Today, 10*(17), 1, 10–12.
Harry Houdini Dies after Operations. (2010, October 31). The *New York Times*. Retrieved from http://www.nytimes.com/learning/general/onthisday/bday/0324.html#top.
Hart, W., Albarracin, D., Eagly, A. H., Brechan, I., Lindberg, M. J., and Merrill, L. (2009). Feeling validated versus being correct: A meta-analysis of selective exposure to information. *Psychological Bulletin, 135*(4), 555–88.
Haswell, R. H. (2005). NCTE/CCCC's recent war on scholarship. *Written Communication, 22,* 198–223. doi: 10.1177/0741088305275367.
Hayhoe, G. F. (2006). Needed research in global technical communication. *Technical Communication, 53,* 141–42.
Healthy People 2020. (2017, February 24). *Health communication and health information technology.* Office of Disease Prevention and Health Promotion. Retrieved from https://www.healthypeople.gov/2020/topics-objectives/topic/health-communication-and-health-information-technology.
Heifferon, B., and Brown, S. C. (2000). Guest editor's column. *Technical Communication Quarterly, 9*(3), 245–48.
Hess, E. (2003). *Yib's guide to MOOing: Getting the most from virtual communities on the Internet*. Retrieved from http://www.lisdude.com/moo/ygm.pdf.
Hine, C. (2005). Research relationships and online relationships: Introduction. In C. Hine (Ed.), *Virtual methods: Issues in social research on the Internet* (pp. 17–20). New York: Berg Publishers.
Hine, C. (2009). Question one: How can qualitative Internet researchers define the boundaries of their projects? In A. N. Markham and N. K. Baym (Eds.), *Internet inquiry: Conversations about method* (pp. 1–20). Thousand Oaks, CA: Sage Publications.
Hinson, K. (2016). Framing illness through Facebook enabled online support groups. *Communication Design Quarterly, 4*(2), 22–32.
Hoover, R. S., and Koerber, A. L. (2011). Using NVivo to answer the challenges of qualitative research in professional communication: Benefits and best practices tutorial. *IEEE Transactions of Professional Communication, 54*.
Huang, G. J., and Penson, D. F. (2008). Internet health resources and the cancer patient. *Cancer Investigation, 26,* 202–7. doi: 10.1080/0735900701566197.
Huckin, T. (2004). Content analysis: What texts talk about. In C. Bazerman and P. Prior (Eds.), *What writing does and how it does it: An introduction to analyzing texts and textual practices* (pp. 13–32). Mahwah, NJ: Lawrence Erlbaum Associates, Inc.
Huffaker, D. (2010). Dimensions of leadership and social influence in online communities. *Health Communication Research, 36,* 593–617. doi: 10.1111/j.1468-2958.2010.01390.x
Hughes, M. A., and Hayhoe, G. F. (2008). *A research primer for technical communication.* New York, NY: Lawrence Erlbaum Associates.
Hwang, K. O., Ottenbacher, A. J., Lucke, J. F., Etchegaray, J. M., Graham, A. L., Thomas, E. J., and Bernstam, E. V. (2011). Measuring social support for weight loss in an Internet weight loss community. *Journal of Health Communication, 16,* 198–211. doi: 10.1080/10810730.2010.535106.
IBM. (n.d.a.). Big data. *IBM big data—What is big data?* Retrieved from http://www.ibm.com/big-data/us/en.
IBM. (n.d.b.). *Dictionary of IBM & computing terminology.* Retrieved from http://www-03.ibm.com/ibm/history/documents/pdf/glossary.pdf.
Ibrahim, Y. (2008). The new risk communities: Social networking sites and risk. *International Journal of Media & Culture Politics, 4,* 244–53.
Im, E.-O., Chee, W., Lim, H.-J., Liu, Y., Guevara, E., and Kim, K. S. (2007). Patients' attitudes toward Internet cancer support groups. *Oncology Nursing Forum, 34*(3), 705–12.

Iriberri, A., and Leroy, G. (2009). A life-cycle perspective on online community success. *ACM Computer Surveys, 41*(2), 11.1–11.29. doi: 10.1145/1459352.1459352.1459356. Retrieved from http://doi.acm.org/10.1145/1459352.1459356.

Ishikawa, H., Hashimoto, H., and Kuichi, T. (2013). The evolving concept of "patient-centeredness" in patient–physician communication research. *Social Science Medicine, 96*, 147–53.

Ji, P., and Lieber, P. S. (2010). Am I safe? Exploring relationships between primary territories and online privacy. *Journal of Internet Commerce, 9,* 3–22. doi: 10.1080/15332861.2010.487413.

Jin, B., Park, J. Y., and Kim, H.-S. (2010). What makes online community members commit? A social exchange perspective. *Behaviour & Information Technology, 29,* 587–99. doi: 10.1080/0144929X.2010.497563.

Johnson, R., and Cureton, A. (2017). Kant's moral philosophy. *The Stanford Encyclopedia of Philosophy*. E. N. Zalta, Ed. Retrieved from https://plato.stanford.edu/archives/spr2017/entries/kant-moral.

Joinson, A. N. (2001). Self-disclosure in computer-mediated communication: The role of self-awareness and visual anonymity. *European Journal of Social Psychology, 31,* 177–92.

Joinson, A. N. (2004). Self-esteem, interpersonal risk, and preference for e-mail to face-to-face communication. *Cyberpsychology & Behavior, 7,* 472–78.

Joinson, A. N., and Dietz-Uhler, B. (2002). Explanations for the perpetration of and reactions to deception in a virtual community. *Social Science Computer Review, 20,* 275–89.

Joinson, A. N., and Paine, C. B. (2007). Chapter 16: Self-disclosure privacy. In A. N. Joinson, K. Y. A. McKenna, T. Postmes, T., and U.-D. Reip, Eds. *The Oxford handbook of Internet psychology* (pp. 237–52).

Jones, Q. (1997). Virtual-communities, virtual settlements & cyber-archaeology: A theoretical outline. *Journal of Computer-Mediated Communication, 3.* Retrieved from http://jcmc.indiana.edu/vol3/issue3/jones.html.

Jones, S. (1999a). Preface. In Jones, S. (Ed.), *Doing Internet research: Critical issues and methods for examining the net* (pp. ix–xiv). Thousand Oaks, CA: SAGE Publications.

Jones, S. (1999b). Studying the net: Intricacies and issues. In Jones, S. (Ed.), *Doing Internet research: Critical issues and methods for examining the net* (pp. 1–27). Thousand Oaks, CA: SAGE Publications.

Jones, V. (2009, October 20). Medical bloggers on ABC New: Empowering patients with accurate information. Retrieved from http://www.youtube.com/watch?v=JARcgVxNkYU.

Kamakshi, P., and Babu, A. V. (2010). Preserving the privacy and sharing the data using classification on perturbed data. *International Journal on Computer Science and Engineering, 2,* 860–64.

Kaminer, D. (2006). Health processes in trauma narratives: A review. *South African Journal of Psychology, 36*(3), 481–99. doi: 10.1177/008124630603600304.

Kastman, L. M., and Gurak, L. J. (1999). Conducting technical communication research via the Internet: Guidelines for privacy, permissions, and ownership in educational research. *Technical Communication, 4,* 460–69.

Kaur, S., and Bawa, R. K. (2015). Future trends of data mining in predicting the various diseases in medical healthcare system. *International Journal of Energy, Information and Communications, 6*(4), 17–34. doi: 10.14257/ijeic.2015.6.4.02 Retrieved from http://www.sersc.org/journals/IJEIC/vol6_Is4/2.pdf.

Kenen, R. H., Shapiro, P. J., Hantsoo, L. Friedman, S., and Coyne, J. C. (2007). Woman with BRCA1 or BRCA2 mutations renegotiating a post-prophylactic mastectomy identity: Self-image and self-disclosure. *Journal of Genetic Counseling, 16,* 789–98. doi: 10.1007/s10897-007-9112-5.

Keränen, L. (2010). Scientific characters: Rhetoric, politics, and trust in breast cancer research. Tuscaloosa, AL: University of Alabama Press.

Kim, J., and Kim, S. (2009). Physicians' perception of the effects of internet health information on the doctor–patient relationship. *Informatics for Health and Social Care, 34*(3), 136–48. doi: 10.1080/17538150903102422

King, C. S. T., Bivens, K., Pumroy, E., Rauch, S., and Koerber, A. (2017). IRB challenges and solutions in health communication research. *Health Communication.* doi: 10.1080/10410236.2017.1321164.

Klitzman, R. (2006). Improving education on doctor–patient relationships and communication: Lessons from doctors who become patients. *Academic Medicine, 81*(5), 447–53.

Koerber, A. (2005). "You just don't see enough normal": Critical perspectives on infant-feeding discourse and practice. *Journal of Business and Technical Communication, 19,* 304–27.

Koerber, A. (2006). Rhetorical agency, resistance, and the disciplinary rhetorics of breastfeeding. *Technical Communication Quarterly, 15,* 87–101.

Koerber, A., and McMichael, L. (2008). Qualitative sampling methods: A primer for technical communicators. *Journal of Business and Technical Communication, 22,* 454–73. doi: 10.1177/1050651908320362.

Koerber, A., and Still, B. (Eds). (2008). Guest editor's introduction: Online health communication. *Technical Communication Quarterly, 17,* 259–63.

Kopelson, K. (2009). Writing patients' wrongs: The rhetoric and reality of information age medicine. *jac: A Journal of Rhetoric, Culture, & Politics, 29*(1–2), 353–404.

Kotowski, M. R., and dos Santos, G. M. (2010). The role of the connector in bridging borders through virtual communities. *Journal of Borderlands Studies, 25*(3–4), 150–58.

Kraetschmer, N., Sharpe, N., Urowitz, S., and Deber, R. B. (2004). How does trust affect patient preferences for participation in decision-making? *Health Expectations, 7,* 317–26.

Krcmar, H., and Leimeister, J. M. (2005). Potentials and benefits of patient communities from a German perspective. *Proceedings of the 11th International Conference on Human-Computer Interaction* (HCI-I 2005), Las Vegas, NV. Retrieved from http://www.uni-kassel.de/fb7/ibwl/leimeister/pub/05-25.pdf.

Kruse, P. (1998). Cybercommunity. *Soujourners, 27*(5), 5.

Kumar, R., Korthius, P. T., Saha, S., Chander, G., Sharp, V., Cohn, J., Moore, R., and Beach, M. C. (2010). Decision-making role preferences among patients with HIV: Associations with patient and provider characteristics and communication behaviors. *Journal of General Internal Medicine, 25*(6), 517–23. doi: 10.1007/s11606-010-1275-3.

Lang, T. (2009). Just who are we and what are we doing, anyway? Needed research in medical writing. *AMWA Journal, 24*(3), 106–12.

Lauzier, S., Maunsell, E., De Koninck, M., Drolet, M., Hebert-Croteau, N., and Robert, J. (2005). Conceptualization and sources of costs from breast cancer: Findings from patient and caregiver focus groups. *Psycho-oncology, 14,* 351–60. doi: 10.1002/pon.851.

Lawson-Tancred, H. C. (2004). Introduction. In Aristotle, *The art of rhetoric* (H. C. Lawson-Tancred, Trans.; pp. 1–61). London, England: Penguin Books. (Original work published 350 BCE).

Lee, D. W., Stang, P. E., Goldberg, G. A., Haberman, M. (2009). Resource use and cost of diagnostic workup of women with suspected breast cancer. *The Breast Journal, 15*(1), 85–92.

Lee, T. S. (2010). DIM (di-indoly methane) for natural protection from estrogen's effects. *NaturoDoc.* Retrieved from http://www.naturodoc.com/library/hormones/diindolymethane.htm.

Leffall, L. D. (1998). Foreword. In K. I. Bland and E. M. Copeland, Eds. *The breast: Comprehensive management of benign and malignant diseases* (p. xvii). Philadelphia, PA: W.B. Saunders Company.

Levin, A., and Abril, P. S. (2009). Two notions of privacy online. *Vanderbilt Journal of Entertainment and Technology Law, 11*(4), 1001–51.

Levine, P. (2002). Building the electronic commons: A project of the Democracy collaborative. *The Good Society, 11*(3), 1–9.

Levinson, W., and Pizzo, P. A. (2011). Patient–physican [*sic*] communication: It's about time. *Journal of the American Medical Association, 305*(17), 1802–3.

Lichtenfeld, L. (2010). *The 2010 statistics are out, and 767,000 people have celebrated more birthdays* [Web log post]. The American Cancer Society. Retrieved from http://www.cancer.

org/AboutUs/DrLensBlog/post/2010/07/07/The-2010-Statistics-Are-Out-And-767000-People-Have-Celebrated-More-Birthdays.aspx.

Lieberman, M.A., and Goldstein, B.A. (2006). Not all negative emotions are equal: The role of emotional expression in online support groups for women with breast cancer. *Psycho-Oncology, 15*, 160–80.

Lissman, T. L., and Boehnlein, J. K. (2001). A critical review of Internet information about depression. *Psychiatric Services, 52*(8), 1046–50.

Liu, G. Z. (1999). Virtual community presence in Internet relay chatting. *Journal of Computer-Mediated Communication, 5*. Retrieved from http://jcmc.indiana.edu/vol2/issue4/mackinnon.html.

Lyne, J. (2001). Contours of intervention: How rhetoric matters to biomedicine, introduction to the special issue on the rhetoric of medicine. Journal of Medical Humanities, 22, 3–13.

MacNealy, M. S. (1999). *Strategies for empirical research in writing.* Needham Heights, MA: Allyn & Bacon.

MacQueen, K. M., McLellan, E., Metzger, D. S., Kegeles, S., Strauss, R., P., Scotti, R., et al. (2001). What is community? An evidence-based definition for participatory public health. *American Journal of Public Health, 91*(12), 1929–38. doi: 10.2105/AJPH.91.12.1929

Main Index—Forum: Gaia Online. (n.d.). *Welcome to Gaia Online*. Retrieved from http://www.gaiaonline.com/forum/index.php.

Maly, R. C., Umezawa, Y., Leake, B., and Silliman, R. A. (2005). Mental health outcomes in older women with breast cancer: Impact of perceived family support and adjustment. *Psycho-Oncology, 14,* 535–45. doi: 10.1002/pon.869.

Manne, S., Ostroff, J., Sherman, M., Glassman, M., Ross, S., Goldstein, L., et al. (2003). Buffering effects of family and friend support on associations between partner unsupportive behaviors and coping among women with breast cancer. *Journal of Social and Personal Relationships, 20,* 771–92.

Marchione, M. (2012, February 25). Cancer's growing burden: The high cost of care. *The Atlanta Journal-Constitution.* Retrieved from http://www.ajc.com/health/cancers-growing-burden-the-1362562.html.

Markman, M., and Luce, R. (2010). Impact of the cost of cancer treatment: An Internet-based survey. *Journal of Oncology Practice, 6*(2), 69–73. doi: 10.1200/JOP.091074

Marr, B. (2014, September 16). Big data: 20 free big data resources everyone should know [Web log]. *SmartData Collective.* Retrieved from http://www.smartdatacollective.com/bernardmarr/235366/big-data-20-free-big-data-sources-everyone-should-know.

Mastectomy Costs. (2010, August 5). *SurgeryCosts.net.* Retrieved from http://www.surgerycosts.net/price.php?medical=mastectomy-

Matzat, U. (2010). Reducing problems of sociability in online communities: Integrating online communication with offline interaction. *American Behavioral Scientist, 53*(8), 1170–93. doi: 10.1177/0002764209356249.

McBride, A. (2005, April 10). Towards a sense of ethics for technical communication. *Orange Journal.* Retrieved http://orange.eserver.org/issues/3-2/mcbride.html

McCabe, J. (2009). Resisting alienation: The social construction of Internet communities supporting eating disorders. *Communication Studies, 60*(1), 1–16.

McCabe, R. M., Adomavicius, G., Johnson, P. E., Ramsey, G., Rund, E., Rush, W. A, et al. (2008). Using data mining to predict errors in chronic disease care. In K. Henriksen, J. B. Battles, M. A. Keyes, and M. L. Grady, Eds., *Advances in patient safety: New directions and alternative approaches* (Vol. 3). Rockville, MD: Agency for Healthcare Research and Quality. Retrieved from https://www.ahrq.gov/downloads/pub/advances2/vol3/Advances-McCabe_39.pdf.

McCullagh, K. (2009). Protecting 'privacy' through control of 'personal' data processing: A flawed approach. *International Review of Law, Computers & Technology, 23*(1–2), 13–24.

McKay, L. (2010). Crafting a community. *Customer Relationships Management,* 24–29.

McKee, H., and Porter, J. E. (2008). The ethics of digital writing research: A rhetorical approach. *College Composition and Communication, 59,* 711–49.

McKee, H. A., and Porter, J. E. (2009). *The ethics of Internet research: A rhetorical, case-based process.* New York: Peter Lang.

McLeod, J., and Wright, K. (2009). The talking cure in everyday life: Gender, generations and friendship. *Sociology, 43,* 122–39. doi:10.1177/0038038508099101.

Medical community. (n.d.). Vocabulary.com. Retrieved from https://www.vocabulary.com/dictionary/medical%20community.

Meloncon, L., and Frost, E. A. (2015). Charting an emerging field: The rhetorics of health and medicine and its importance in communication design. *Communication Design Quarterly Review, 3*(4), 7–14.

Merry, S. K., and Simon, A. (2012). Living and lurking on LiveJournal: The benefits of active and non-active membership. *Aslib Proceedings, 64*(3), 241–61. doi: 10.1108/00012531211244527.

Milson, A. J., and Chu, B-W. (2002). Character education for cyberspace: Developing good netizens. *The Social Studies,* 117–19.

Mohamed, A. A.-A. (2010). Online privacy concerns among social networks' users. *Cross-Cultural Communication, 6*(4), 74–89.

Mol, A. (2002). *The body multiple: Ontology in medical practice.* Durham, NC: Duke University Press.

Mooney, G., and Ryan, M. (2003). Agency in health care: Getting beyond first principles. *Journal of Health Economics, 12,* 125–35.

Moore, M. G. (1993). Theory of transactional distance. In D. Keegan (Ed.), *Theoretical principles of distance education* (pp. 22–39). New York: Routledge.

Morgan, M. A. (2009, February). Considering the patient–partner relationship in cancer care: Coping strategies for couples. *Clinical Journal of Oncology Nursing, 13*(1), 65–72.

Moulton, B., and King, J. S. (2010). Aligning ethics with medical decision-making: The quest for informed patient choice. *The Effects of Health Information Technology on the Physician–Patient Relationship*, 85–97.

Mulcahy, N. (2013, April 25). New adverse event in cancer treatment; "Financial toxicity" [Online]. *Medscape Medical News.* Retrieved from http://www.medscape.com/viewarticle/803111.

Muller, A. (2016). Get satisfaction community rules. *Get satisfaction.* Retrieved from http://getsatisfaction.com/help/community-guidelines.

Nah, S. (2010). A theoretical and analytical framework toward networked communities: A case of the electronic community information commons. *Javahost—The Public, 17*(1), 23–36.

National Breast Cancer Foundation, Inc. (2016). *Male breast cancer*. Retrieved from http://www.nationalbreastcancer.org/male-breast-cancer.

National Cancer Institute. (n.d.a.) *Cancer Stat Facts: Female Breast Cancer.* Retrieved from https://seer.cancer.gov/statfacts/html/breast.html.

National Cancer Institute. (n.d.b.). *Comprehensive cancer information—Probability of breast cancer in American women*. Retrieved from http://www.cancer.gov/cancertopics/factsheet/detection/probability-breast-cancer.

National Institutes of Health. (n.d.). *Training: Protection of human research participants.* Retrieved from https://phrp.nihtraining.com/index.php.

Nierengarten, M. B. (2005, December). *Nonanthracycline TC adjuvant chemo superior for operable breast cancer* [abstract]. Paper presented at the 28th Annual San Antonio Breast Cancer Symposium, San Antonio, TX. Retrieved from http://www.medscape.com/viewarticle/519565.

Noddings, N. (2012). The language of care ethics. *Knowledge Quest, 40*(4), 52–56.

Obst, P., and Stafurik, J. (2010). Short research note: Online we are all able bodied: Online psychological sense of community and social support found through membership of disability-specific Websites promotes well-being for people living with a physical disability *Journal of Community & Applied Social Psychology, 20,* 525–31. doi: 10.1002/casp.1067.

O'Connor, B., and Mackeogh, C. (2007). New media communities: Performing identity in an online women's magazine. *Irish Journal of Sociology, 16*(2), 97–116.

Oettel, M., and Mukhopadhyay, A. K. (2004). Progesterone: The forgotten hormone in men? *The Aging Male, 7,* 236–57. doi: 10.1080/13685530400004199.

O'Hair, D., Villagran, M. M., Wittenberg, E., et al. (2003). Cancer survivorship and agency model: Implications for patient choice, decision making, and influence. *Health Communication, 15,* 193–202.

OHSR. (n.d.) *Office of Human Subjects Research Belmont Report guidelines*. Retrieved from http://ohsr.od.nih.gov/guidelines/belmont.html

Oppegaard, B. (2015). "Future of media: A mobile mindset." In C. S. Lambert and M. Schlobohm, *Communication and emerging media: What's trending now*. Dubuque, IA: Kendall Hunt Publishers.

Orgad, S. (2006). The cultural dimensions of online communication: A study of breast cancer patients' Internet spaces. *New Media & Society, 8*(6), 877–99. doi: 10.1177/1461444806069643.

Owen, J. E., Bantum, E. O., and Golant, M. (2009). Benefits and challenges experienced by professional facilitators of online support groups for cancer survivors. *Psycho-Oncology, 18,* 144–55.

Owens, K. H. (2011). Rhetorics of e-Health and information age medicine: A risk-benefit analysis. *JAC: A Journal of Rhetoric, Culture, & Politics,* 31(1–2), 225–34.

Paternotte E, van Dulmen S, van der Lee N, Scherpbier AJJA, Scheele F. Factors influencing intercultural doctor–patient communication: A realistic review. *Patient Ed Counsel.* 2015; 98: 420–45.

Peck, M. S. (1987). The different drum: Community making and peace. New York, NY: Touchstone.

Pennebaker, J. W. (1990). *Opening up: The healing power of confiding in others.* New York: William Morrow and Company, Inc.

Pennebaker, J. W. (1993). Putting stress into words: Health, linguistic and therapeutic implications. *Behavior Research & Therapy, 31,* 539–48.

Pennebaker, J. W., and Seagal, J. D. (1999). Forming a story: The health benefits of narrative. *Journal of Clinical Psychology, 55*(10), 1243–54.

Pennebaker, J. W., Kiecolt-Glaser, J. K., and Glaser, R. (1988). Disclosure of traumas and immune function: Health implications for psychotherapy. *Journal of Consulting & Clinical Psychology, 56,* 239–45.

Pennebaker, J. W., and Susman, J. R. (1988). Disclosure of traumas and psychosomatic processes. *Social Science & Medicine, 26,* 327–32.

Pezzullo, P. C. (2003). Resisting "National Breast Cancer Awareness Month": The rhetoric of counterpublics and their cultural performances. *Quarterly Journal of Speech, 89*(4), 345–65.

Pitts, V. (2004). Illness and Internet empowerment: Writing and reading breast cancer in cyberspace. *Health, 8*(1), 33–59. doi: 10.117/1363459304038794.

Present Tense Editors. (2012, October 21). Special double issue on medical, gender, and body rhetorics. *Present Tense,* 1–2. Retrieved from http://www.presenttensejournal.org/editorial/vol-2-2-issue-introduction.

Propinquity. (n.d.). *Merriam-Webster dictionary.* Retrieved from http://www.merriam-webster.com/dictionary/propinquity.

PubMed Health. (n.d.). Docetaxel injection. *National Center for Biotechnology information.* Retrieved from http://www.ncbi.nlm.nih.gov/pubmedhealth/PMH0000987.

PubMed Health. (2011). Zoledronic acid injection. *National Center for Biotechnology information.* Retrieved from http://www.ncbi.nlm.nih.gov/pubmedhealth/PMH0000306.

QSR International. (2010). NVivo 9 Basics. ABN, Australia: QSR International Pty Ltd.

Radin, P. (2006). "To me, it's my life": Medical communication, trust, and activism in cyberspace. *Social Science & Medicine, 62,* 591–601. doi: 10.1016/j.socscimed.2005.06.022.

Rakower, L. H. (2011). Blurred line: Zooming in on Google street view and the global right to privacy. *Brooklyn Journal of International Law, 37,* (317–47).

Ravdin, P. M., Cronin, K. A., Howlader, N., Berg, C. D., Chlebowski, R. T., Fuerer, E. J., et al. (2007). Special report: The decrease in breast-cancer incidence in 2003 in the United States. *New England Journal of Medicine, 356,* 1670–74. doi: 10.1056/NEJMsr070105.

Reich, S. M. (2010). Adolescents' sense of community on MySpace and Facebook: A mixed-methods approach. *Journal of Community Psychology, 38,* 688–705. doi: 10.1002/jcop.20389.

Remler, D. K., and Van Ryzin, G. G. (2011). *Research methods in practice: Strategies for description and causation.* Los Angeles, CA: Sage Publications.

Rheingold, H. (1993). *The virtual community: Homesteading on the electronic frontier.* Reading, MA: Addison-Wesley.

Riding, C., Gefen, D., and Arinze, B. (2006). Psychological barriers: Lurker and poster motivation and behavior in online communities. *Communications of the Association for Information Systems, 18,* 329–54.

Roberts. (1999). A rape in cyberspace. *CS181 Controlling the Virtual World.* Retrieved from https://cs.stanford.edu/people/eroberts/cs181/projects/1998-99/controlling-the-virtual-world/history/rape.html.

Roberts, C., and Sarangi, S. (2005). Theme-oriented discourse analysis of medical encounters. *Medical Education, 39,* 632–40.

Robins, K. (2007). Against virtual community: For a politics of distance. In D. Bell and B. M. Kennedy (Eds.), *The cybercultures reader* (2nd ed.) (pp. 227–35). London, UK: Routledge.

Rodgers, S., and Chen, Q. (2005). Internet community group participation: Psychosocial benefits for women with breast cancer. *Journal of Computer-Mediated Communication, 10.* Retrieved from http://jcmc.indiania.edu/vol10/issue4/rodgers.html.

Rose, J. H. (1990). Social support and cancer: Adult patients' desire for support from family, friends, and health professionals. *American Journal of Community Psychology, 18,* 439–64.

Rude, C. D. (2012, May). How can technical communication academics and practitioners develop research relationships, and why should we care? Presentation at Texas Tech University's TCR May Seminar, Lubbock, TX.

Rutter, J., and Smith, G. W. H. (2005). Ethnographic presence in a nebulous setting. In C. Hine (Ed.), *Virtual methods: Issues in social research on the Internet* (pp. 81–92). New York: Berg Publishers.

Ryan, C. (2017). History of communication and media. In C. S. Lambert and M. Schlobohm, *Communication and emerging media: What's trending now* (pp. 1–26). Dubuque, IA: Kendall Hunt.

Saint-Jacques, N., Younis, T., Dewar, R., and Rayson, D. (2007). Wait times for breast cancer care. *British Journal of Cancer, 96,* 162–68.

Samant, R., Aivas, I., Bourque, J.-M., and Tucker, T. (2010). Oncology residents' perspectives on communication skills and shared decision making. *Journal of Cancer Education, 25,* 474–77. doi: 10.1007/s13187-010-0094-x.

SAS Institute Inc. (n.d.). Health analytics: What it is and why it matters. *Health Analytics—SAS.* Retrieved from https://www.sas.com/en_us/insights/health-analytics.html.

Schryer, C. F., Lingard, L., Spafford, M., and Garwood, K. (2003). Structure and agency in medical case presentations. In C. Bazerman and D. Russell (Eds.), *Writing selves/writing societies: Research from activity perspectives.* Fort Collins, CO: WAC Clearinghouse and Mind, Culture, and Activity. Retrieved from http://wac.colostate.edu/books/selves_societies.

Scott, B., Segal, J. Z., and Keränen, L. (2013). The rhetorics of health and medicine: Inventional possibilities for scholarship and engaged practice. *Poroi: An Interdisciplinary Journal of Rhetorical Analysis and Invention, 9*(1), doi: 10.13008/2151-2957.1157.

Seattle Cancer Care Alliance. (2017). About breast prosthetics & mastectomy bras. Retrieved from https://www.seattlecca.org/shine/oncology-products/breast-prostheses-and-bras/about-breast-prosthetics-mastectomy-bras.

Segal, J. Z. (2005). *Health and the rhetoric of medicine.* Carbondale, IL: Southern Illinois University Press.

Segal, J. Z. (2009). Internet health and the 21st-century patient: A rhetorical view. *Written Communication, 26,* 351–69.

Seigel, M. (2013). The rhetoric of pregnancy. Chicago, IL: University of Chicago Press.

Sharf, B. F. (1997). Communicating breast cancer on-line: Support and empowerment on the Internet. *Women & Health, 26*(1), 65–84.

Shipman, B. (2010). The role of communication in the patient–physician relationship. *The Journal of Legal Medicine, 31,* 433–42. doi: 10.1080/10947648.2010.535427.

Shah, S. G. S., and Robinson, I. (2011). Patients' perspectives on self-testing of oral anticoagulation therapy: Content analysis of patients' internet blogs. *BMC Health Services Research, 11*(25). doi: 10.1186/1472-6963-11-25.

Shen, K. N., Yu, A. Y., and Khalifa, M. (2010). Knowledge contribution in virtual communities: Accounting for multiple dimensions of social presence through social identity. *Behaviour & Information Technology, 29*(4), 337–48.

Sidler, M., and Jones, N. (2009). Genetics interfaces: Representing science and enacting public discourse in online spaces. *Technical Communication Quarterly, 18,* 28–48. doi: 10.10.1080/10572250802437317.

Silver, N. (2012). *The signal and the noise.* New York, NY: Penguin Press.

Singer, M. G. (2003). Nineteenth-century British ethics. In L. C. Becker and C. B. Becker, Eds., *A history of Western ethics* (pp. 95–113). New York: Routledge.

Singer, N. (2012, November 11). When a palm reader knows more than your life line. *The New York Times.* Retrieved from http://www.nytimes.com/2012/11/11/technology/biometric-data-gathering-sets-off-a-privacy-debate.html?module=ArrowsNav&contentCollection=Technology&action=keypress&region=FixedLeft&pgtype=article.

Slanina, F., and Konopásek, Z. (2010). Eigenvector localization as a tool to study small communities in online social networks. *Advances in Complex Systems, 13*(6), 699–723. doi: 10.1142/S0219525910002840.

Smith, C., Guyton, K., Pariser, J. J., Siegler, M., Schindler, N., and Langerman, A. (2016). Surgeon–patient communication during awake procedures. *American Journal of Surgery.* doi: 10.1016/j.amjsurg.2016.06.017

Srinivasan, M. (2011). From the editor's desk: Hippocrates and patient-centered medicine. *Journal of General Internal Medicine, 27*(2), 135. doi: 10.1007/s11106-011-1948-6.

Steinberg, G. B., Church, B. W., McCall, C. J., Scott, A. B., and Kalis, B. P. (2014). Novel predictive models for metabolic syndrome risk: A big data analytic approach. *American Journal of Managed Care, 20*(6), e221–e228. Retrieved from http://www.ajmc.com/journals/issue/2014/2014-vol20-n6/Novel-Predictive-Models-for-Metabolic-Syndrome-Risk-A-Big-Data-Analytic-Approach#sthash.2HsLwB6k.dpuf.

Steinmetz, K. F. (2012). Message received: Virtual ethnography in online message boards. *International Journal of Qualitative Research, 11*(1), 26–39.

Stewart, T. (2010). Editorial: Online communities. *Behaviour & Information Technology, 29*(6), 555–56.

Still, B. (2008). *Online intersex communities: Virtual neighborhoods of support and activism.* Amherst, NY: Cambria Press.

Street, R. L., and Voigt, B. (1997). Patient participation in deciding breast cancer treatment and subsequent quality of life. *Medical Decision Making, 17*(3), 298–306. doi: 10.1177/0272989X9701700306.

Suler, J. (2004). The online disinhibition effect. *CyberPsychology & Behavior, 7*(3), 321–26.

Sundar, S. S., and Marathe, S. S. (2010). Personalization versus customization: The importance of agency, privacy, and power usage. *Human Communication Research, 36,* 298–322. doi: 10.1111/j.1468-2958.2010.01377.x.

Swenson, S. L., Buell, S., Zettler, P., White, M., Ruston, D. C., and Lo, B. (2004). Patient-centered communication: Do patients really prefer it? *Journal of General Internal Medicine, 19,* 1069–79.

Szabo, L. (2008, October 13). Cancer patients forgoing care because of cost; Many face hard choices. *USA Today,* 5D.

Talen, M. R., Grampp, K., Tucker, A., and Schultz, J. (2008). What physicians want from their patients: Identifying what makes good patient communication. *Families, Systems, & Health, 26,* 58–66.

Tang, S. Y. S., and Anderson, J. M. (1999). Human agency and the process of healing: Lessons learned from women living with a chronic illness—'re-writing the expert.' *Nursing Inquiry, 6,* 83–93.

Tann, J., Platts, A., Welch, S., and Allen, J. (2003). Patient power? Medical perspectives on patient use of the Internet. *Prometheus: Critical Studies in Innovation, 21*(2), 145–60. doi: 10.1080/08109020308131.

Tene, O. (2008). What Google knows: Privacy and Internet search engines. *Utah Law Review, 4,* 1433–92.

Thom, D. H. (2001). Physician behaviors that predict patient trust. *The Journal of Family Practice, 50,* 323–28.

Thomas, F., Aggleton, P., and Anderson, J. (2010). 'Experts,' 'partners' and 'fools': Exploring agency in HIV treatment seeking among African migrants in London. *Social Science & Medicine*, 70, 736–43. doi: 10.1016/j.socscimed.2009.10.063.

Throsby, K. (2007). "How could you let yourself get like that?": Stories of the origins of obesity in accounts of weight loss surgery. *Social Science & Medicine, 65*, 1561–71. doi:10.1016/j.socscimed.2007.06.005.

Tiedtke, C., de Rijk, A., de Casterle, B. D., Christiaens, M., and Donceel, P. (2010). Experiences and concerns about 'returning to work' for women breast cancer survivors: A literature review. *Psycho-Oncology, 19,* 677–83.

Traumatic. (n.d.). *The Free Dictionary*. Retrieved from http://www.thefreedictionary.com/traumatic.

Tsai, M.-H., Lu, F.-H., and Frankel, R. M. (2013). Learning to listen: Effects of using conversational transcripts to help medical students improve their use of open questions in soliciting patient problems. *Patient Ed Counseling, 93,* 48–55.

Tucker, S. (2012). *Journey through the storm: A faith walk through cancer.* Dallas, TX: Cross House Publishing.

Turner, B. S. (2009). Citizens, communities and conflicts: Surviving globalization. *Citizenship Studies, 13,* 431–37.

U.S. Department of Homeland Security. (2009, March 19). Testimony of Deputy Assistant Secretary for Policy Kathleen Kraninger, screening coordination, and Director Robert A. Mocny, US-VISIT, National Protection and Programs Directorate, before the House Appropriations Committee, Subcommittee on Homeland Security, "biometric identification." *Testimony on Biometric Identification—Homeland Security.* Retrieved from https://www.dhs.gov/news/2009/03/19/testimony-biometric-identification.

Vera-Llonch, M., Weycker, D., Glass, A., Gao, S., Borker, R., Qin, A., and Oster, G. (2011). Healthcare costs in women with metastatic breast cancer receiving chemotherapy as their principal treatment modality. *BMC Cancer 11*, 250. Retrieved from http://bmccancer.biomedcentral.com/articles/10.1186/1471-2407-11-250. doi: 10.1186/1471-2407-11-250.

Wagner, F. B., Martin, R. G., and Bland, K. I. (1998). History of the therapy of breast disease. In K. I. Bland and E. M. Copeland, Eds. *The breast: Comprehensive management of benign and malignant diseases* (pp. 1–18). Philadelphia, PA: W.B. Saunders Company.

Walker, B. (2015, April 5). Every day big data statistics—2.5 quintillion bytes of data created daily [infographic]. *VCloud News.* Retrieved from http://www.vcloudnews.com/every-day-big-data-statistics-2-5-quintillion-bytes-of-data-created-daily.

Walmsley, D. J. (2000). Community, Place and Cyberspace. *Australian Geographer, 31*(1), 5–19.

Want, E. S.-T., Chen, L. S.-L., and Tsai, B.-K. (2012). Emerald article: Investigating member commitment to virtual communities using an integrated perspective. *Internet Research, 22*(2), 199–210. doi: 10.1108/10662241211214566.

WebMD LLC. (2016). Be part of the WebMD community. Retrieved from http://exchanges.webmd.com/default.htm.

Welcome—Gaia Online. (2016). *About Gaia Online.* Retrieved from http://www.gaiaonline.com.

Wellman, B., and Gulia, M. (1997). Net surfers don't ride alone: Virtual communities as communities. In P. Kollock and M. Smith (Eds.), *Communities and cyberspace*. New York: Routledge.

Wenger, E. (2006, June). Communities of practice: A brief introduction. Retrieved from www.ewenger.com/theory.

West, R. E. (2010). A student's guide to strengthening an online community. *TechTrends, 54*(5), 69–77.

"What is breast cancer?" (2017). *Breastcancer.org*. Retrieved from http://www.breastcancer.org/symptoms/understand_bc/what_is_bc.

"What units of measurement are used for data storage?" (2012, October 13). *TechTerms.* Retrieved from https://techterms.com/help/data_storage_units_of_measurement.

"What's a Byte." (2017). *Megabytes, gigabytes, terabytes . . . What are they?* Retrieved from http://whatsabyte.com.

Whilock, J. L., Powers, J. L., and Eckenrode, J. (2006). The virtual cutting edge: The Internet and adolescent self-injury. *Developmental Psychology, 42,* 407–17. doi: 10.1037/0012-1649.42.3.407.

White-Farnham, J., Finer, B. S., and Molloy, C. (2017). *Call for chapter proposals for an edited collection—Women, patient, advocate: 21 st century women's health rhetorics.*

Whitehouse, G. (2010). Newsgathering and privacy: Expanding ethics codes to reflect change in the digital media age. *Journal of Mass Media Ethics, 25,* 310–27. doi: 10.1080/08900523.2010.512827.

Whitten, P., Smith, S., Munday, S., and LaPlante, C. (2008). Communication assessment of the most frequented breast cancer websites: Evaluation of design and theoretical criteria. *Journal of Computer-Mediated Communication, 13,* 880–911.

Whitty, M. T., and Joinson, A. N. (2009). *Truth, lies and trust on the Internet.* New York: Psychology Press.

Wilce, J. M. (2009). Medical discourse. *Annual Review of Anthropology, 38*, 199–215.

Windsor, D. (2006). Using writing to structure agency: An examination of engineers' practice. *Technical Communication Quarterly, 15,* 411–30.

Woods, C. S. (2013). Repunctuated feminism: Marketing menstrual suppression through the rhetoric of choice. *Women's Studies in Communication, 32*, 267–87. doi: 10.1080/07491409.2013.829791.

Xia, M., Huang, Y., Duan, W., and Whinston, A. B. (2009). Ballot Box communication in online communities. *Communications of the ACM, 52*(9), 138–42. doi: 10.1145/1562164.1562199.

Yahoo View. (2017, June 16). JetBlue tests facial recognition technology. *Yahoo!News.* Retrieved from https://www.yahoo.com/news/jetblue-tests-facial-recognition-technology-154728774.html.

Yee, N., and Bailenson, J. (2007). The Proteus effect: The effect of transformed self-representation on behavior. *Human Communication Research, 33,* 271–90. doi: 10.1111/j.1468-2958-2007-00299.x.

Yeh, N.-C., Lin, J. C.-C., and Lu, H.-P. (2011). The moderating effect of social roles on user behaviour in virtual worlds. *Online Information Review, 35,* 747–69. doi: 10.1108/14684521111176480.

Young, J. R. (2001). Committee of scholars proposes ethics guidelines for research in cyberspace. *Chronicle of Higher Education, 48*(10), A51.

Zabinski, M. F., Celio, A. A., Jacobs, M. J., Manwaring, J., and Wilfley, D. E. (2003). Internet-based prevention of eating disorders. *European Eating Disorders Review, 11,* 183–97. doi: 10.1002/erv.525.

Zancheti, S. M. (2002). Values, built heritage and cyberspace. *Museum International, 54*(3), 19–31.

Zaugg, H., West, R. E., Tateishi, I., and Randall, D. L. (2011). Mendeley: Creating communities of scholarly inquiry through research collaboration. *TechTrends, 55*(1), 32–36.

Zhang, B. (2017, May 15). Delta wants to use facial recognition technology to make checking your bags easier. *Business Insider.* Retrieved from http://www.businessinsider.com/delta-facial-recognition-software-check-bag-lines-2017-5.

Zun, L. S., Blume, D. N., Lester, J., Simpson, G., and Downey, L. (2004). Accuracy of emergency medical information on the Web. *American Journal of Emergency Medicine, 22*(2), 94–97. doi: 10.1016/j.ajem.2003.12.009.

Zun, L., Downey, L., and Brown, S. (2011). Completeness and accuracy of emergency medical information on the Web: Update 2008. *Western Journal of Emergency Medicine, 12*(4). Retrieved from http://escholarship.org/uc/item/5tw9818k.

Index

About the Author

Carie S. Tucker King is clinical professor of communication and associate director of rhetoric at The University of Texas at Dallas. She has a Bachelor of Arts in English from Baylor University, a Master of Arts in Technical Writing from the University of North Texas, and a Doctorate of Philosophy in Technical Communication and Rhetoric from Texas Tech University. She also completed additional graduate coursework in communication, ethics, and medicine through the Center for Spirituality and Ethics at the Texas Tech University Health Sciences Center. Previously, she was a medical editor and communication consultant to physicians and researchers in various U.S. medical schools. Now, she teaches communication, ethics, advanced writing, and research courses for students pursuing degrees in art and technology, humanities, engineering, computer science, and premedical fields. She loves to work with students and to research online patient discourse as well as STEM writing. She lives north of Dallas with her husband David and three of their five children.

www.ingramcontent.com/pod-product-compliance
Ingram Content Group UK Ltd.
Pitfield, Milton Keynes, MK11 3LW, UK
UKHW040153091026
15587UKWH00018B/133

9 781498 552448